ELIXIR
of the
AGELESS
YOU ARE WHAT YOU DRINK

THE HEALING POWER OF LIQUID
CRYSTAL WATER

ELECTRO-COLLOIDAL MINERAL
CONCENTRATE

BY

DR. G. PATRICK FLANAGAN
Ph.D., M.D. (M.A.)
GAEL CRYSTAL FLANAGAN
M.D. (M.A.)

EDITED BY

JOSEPH ANDREW MARCELLO

This edition published by CreateSpace

ISBN 10: 1533074364

ISBN 13: 978-1533074362

Table of Contents

APPENDIX

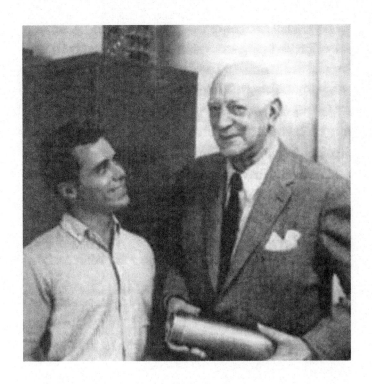

Dr. Patrick Flanagan and Dr. Henri Coanda

Dr. Henri Coanda, the Father of Fluid Dynamics, and Patrick Flanagan at Huyck Research Laboratories in Stamford, Connecticut in June, 1965.

Dr. Coanda was the scientist who discovered that the secret of long life was in the structure of water. He told Patrick, "We are what we drink."

Dr. Coanda gave Patrick the secrets of a lifetime of water research, and started Patrick on his quest for the secret of Hunza water.

This photograph was taken by astrophysicist G. Harry Stine.

CHAPTER 1

THE ELIXIR OF THE AGELESS

High in the mountains of northern India, in the foothills of the Hindu Kush lies the legendary Shangri La. The movie *Lost Horizon* was filmed in the area of the small country known as Hunza.

In the film, Shangri La was a high altitude hidden valley surrounded by jagged mountain peaks.

The people of Shangri La lived in an age-less condition as long as they stayed in their valley which had the power to bestow eternal youth upon those who lived there.

Although Shangri La is just a legend, most legends have some basis in fact. In the rugged land of Hunza, people have lifespans of up to 130 years and enjoy excellent health free of the diseases that ravage modern man. In fact, many of these people have children after the age of 100!

The trek to Hunzaland is treacherous. As the traveler leaves Shrinagar he climbs high into the Karakorum mountains using narrow trails that cling perilously to rocky slopes. He crosses hanging rope bridges that span chasms dropping 3,000 feet to icy rivers.

Eventually he reaches the 8,000 foot mountain valley which is Hunzaland. This hidden valley is surrounded by over 100 mountains that rise above 20,000 feet.

These mountain peaks with blue glaciers are millions of years old. In the distance he can see the peak of Nanga Parbat the third highest mountain in the world.

Through decades, dozens of scientists and health investigators have made the trek to Hunza in an effort to unlock the secrets of long life and eternal youth.

Most investigators have studied the Hunza diet, (believing the secret of long life was in what these people ate.) While diet is extremely important, the first Hunza secret is not in what they eat, but in what they drink. They believe their water is an elixir of long life.

The Mir or King of Hunza told health researcher Betty Lee Morales: "Our good health and long life is in our water. It comes from the glaciers and carries with it special minerals that revitalize our cells."

Throughout history hundreds of explorers have traveled the world in search of a legendary 'Fountain of Youth.' Could it be that this fountain lies in the remote region of Hunza?

Actually, there are at least five areas on Earth where people live to be in excess of 100. These areas have one thing in common--the people of these places claim that the special cloudy minerals in their water keep them young and healthy.

In all cases, the water is cloudy, and comes from ice blue glaciers. Glacier water has no minerals and is nearly identical in composition to distilled water. In springtime, as the glacier melts, water travels through special mineral beds and absorbs high energy colloidal minerals in its journey.

In the early 1930's, Dr. Henri Coanda, a Rumanian Scientist who is known in our time as the 'Father of Fluid Dynamics' made the arduous journey to Hunza.

Coanda also traveled to the five other remote areas on Earth where people live to be over 100 and remain in perfect health.

The areas Dr. Coanda had visited included the county of Georgia high in the mountains of Russia, a remote community in outer Mongolia, the Vilcabamba mountain valley in Ecuador, and a hidden valley in Peru.

In each of these places the natives attribute their health and long life to their precious cloudy colloidal mineral water.

As a result of these investigations Dr. Coanda came to the conclusion that the old saying: "We are what we eat" should be changed to "We are what we drink." Coanda spent most of his long life in search of the secret of Hunza water. When he died he was the president of the Rumanian Academy of Sciences.

In the early 1960's, Dr. Coanda was hired as a consultant by Huyck Research Laboratories in Stamford, Connecticut. Huyck Corporation, had developed a think tank that was involved in far reaching research into unusual scientific phenomena.

Huyck labs was investigating two major research projects at the time, the Coanda Effect and an electronic hearing device of my invention which was known as the Neurophone. I was 18 years old and Dr. Coanda was nearing 75.

The Coanda Effect is the phenomenon of fluid flow that enables airplanes to fly. Simply stated, when a fluid flows over a surface it tends to cling to that surface.

If the surface curves the fluid will follow the curve and will also entrain or capture outside fluid along with it. If the curve and the fluid flow are in resonance with each other, the device will act as a fluid amplifier, that is it will increase flow volume and/or acceleration.

This discovery led to the development of fluid computers, fluid amplifiers and a variety of other inventions to make life easier.

One of his Coanda Effect inventions produces such a rapid change in fluid flow and pressure that it reduces the temperature of air flowing over the surfaces. This change is so great that if water is injected into the air flow it produces ice crystals and perfect snowflakes. This device is called a Coanda Nozzle.

In the 1930's he used the device to make the first artificial snow for the ski slopes of France.

While at Huyck Labs, Coanda was assisting in the development of a number of devices that utilized the Coanda Effect. These included a torpedo that could travel through water at 100 miles per hour without creating a wake.

On Coanda's 75th birthday a party was thrown in his honor at the New Canaan home of G. Harry Stine, Director of Research at the laboratory. As I was 18 years old, I wanted to say something complimentary to Coanda.

So I told him that I hoped that I would be in as good health as he was when I was 75 years old. Coanda looked me in the eye and said, "When you are 75 Years old, Patrick, we will talk about it."

As Coanda and I were both inventors and consultants at Huyck we became good friends. One day Dr. Coanda asked me to come into his office for a visit. He told me he wanted to tell me something of great importance.

He said he wanted to share the results of his lifelong search for the Fountain of Youth. Since he would probably not complete his research, he thought I might discover the answer since I had my entire life ahead of me.

He told me about his world travels during which he had examined the precious glacier waters of Hunza, the county Georgia in Russia, the high mountain valleys of Mongolia and the Andes and Peru, but he had not deciphered the secret of these waters.

He explained that the secret of lot was somehow related to the molecular structure of water. He was able to test waters in these places by turning samples into snowflakes by using his snowmaking fluid amplifier.

He said that snowflakes are living forms with a circulatory system composed of tiny tubes in the center of the snowflake structure. These tubes are an analog of the circulatory systems in animals and plants. They are tiny veins that circulate water that is not yet frozen.

This water is anomalous water, that is, the venous liquid crystal water of the snowflake does not freeze at zero Celsius like ordinary water. It freezes much more slowly. When the water in these veins does eventually freeze the snowflake is dead.

By timing the life of the snowflake he was able to establish a direct relationhip to the human lifespan in the area where the water was tested. He said this anomalous water was the key to the long life of the Hunza people.

He said that he believed I would someday discover the secret of the cause of this anomaly and as a result I would be able to give the benefits of Hunza water to people all over world. That was in 1963; shortly after that I went back to my home in Bellaire, Texas and Dr. Henri Coanda went to Rumania where he became the president of the Rumanian Academy of Sciences.

CHAPTER 2

SEARCH FOR THE SECRET OF
THE FOUNTAIN OF YOUTH

The meeting with Dr. Coanda marked the beginning of a 24-year search for the secret of Hunza water.

It seems that water is an elusive substance whose real structure evades identity. To this day (August 1986) no one in the world really knows what the structure of liquid water really is; however, we do know that it does have structure.

Bulk water found in lakes, streams and oceans is a sea of chaos that has very little structure. However, X-Ray diffraction studies show that within this sea of chaos are a small percentage of molecules that are liquid crystals. This percentage changes with temperature. These liquid crystals may be considered as 'icebergs' floating in a random sea of violent molecular motion. These structures exist at all temperatures, even in boiling water. As water approaches the freezing point the number of liquid crystals increases.

We do know the basic formula for water is H-O-H or H_2O. This formula is only true for water in pure vapor form. The moment we condense water vapor into a liquid form its formula becomes more complex.

It might be said that water contains liquid crystals of variable bonding. This means that water may change structure depending on the effects of internal or external energy fields.

Its structure changes according to the composition of containers that hold it. Water can hold varying proportions of gases dissolved into its structure, the most common being carbon dioxide, nitrogen and oxygen.

Water is the primordial substance in which all life gives birth, and from which all life is sustained. It is indeed an unusual substance.

Water covers three fourths of the Earth's surface, and makes up an average of 71% of our entire body weight. Our muscles are composed of 75% water, our brains are composed of 90% water, the liver is 69% water, and our bones are 22% water.

In the same way that water is not evenly distributed in the body, the water of the Earth is not evenly distributed over its surface.

Most of the Earth's water is held in ocean basins in a form that is unsuitable for drinking or irrigation of crops.

The only time water is suitable for plant and animal use is when it is distilled by nature into, pure, mineral-free form, at which time it falls as rain in varying amounts from place to place and time to time.

In the same way the water evaporates from the oceans only to fall back to the land, our bodily water evaporates and flows from the surface of the body, it is breathed out with every breath, and it must be continuously replaced in order for us to remain alive.

We pour approximately five times our body weight down our throats every year, and by the time we die we drink about 7,000 gallons or 56,000 pounds of it.

Pure drinking water is so rare that throughout history we can write the story of man's growth in terms of his epic concern for it.

Water is the only substance on Earth that is simultaneously available in three distinct states: solid, liquid, and gaseous.

In chemistry and physics, these three states of matter are known as phases. The state of each phase is dependent upon the temperature of the substance.

Most substances can be made to assume one or more of the three forms by manipulating its temperate environment.

Since the basic formula for the individual water molecule is H_2O, which means that an individual molecule consists of two atoms of hydrogen bound to one molecule of oxygen, it is structure to other materials like H_2Te (Te for tellurium), H_2Se (Se for selenium), and H_2S (S for sulfur).

If we examine these substances from physical point of view, following known laws of substances, we would expect these substances to follow certain rules.

That is, the boiling and freezing points of these substances should follow the rule that the lightest of these being water should have the lowest freezing and boiling points, and that the heaviest of these should have the highest. As it turns out, three of the substances do follow the rule.

H_2Te with a molecular weight of 129 boils at -4°C, and freezes at -51°C. H_2Se with a molecular weight of 80 boils at -42°C., and freezes at -64°C. H_2S at a weight of 34 boils at - 61°C., and freezes at -62°C.

On this scale, the predicted points of water at a molecular weight of 18 should be -100°C. for freezing and 80°C. for boiling!

We all know from basic chemistry that water at sea level freezes at 0°C. and boils at 100°C. Now we begin to see that water is indeed an unusual substance.

We know that when water is cooled toward the freezing point, it begins to contract. That is, its density increases to 4°C. (39°F). At this temperature, which is right above freezing, water reaches its maximum density.

As it is cooled the other four degrees to freezing, it does a strange thing; it expands. Water expands a full 10% at the point at which it becomes ice. Because of this expansion, ice is lighter than water and floats. If this expansion did not occur, ice would form on the bottom of a lake first, and would kill the life forms that live there.

Water exhibits a force know as surface tension. Surface tension is the force that causes water to stick to itself or pull itself together. It is surface tension that causes rain drops to assume a spherical shape, the sphere being the only shape that requires the least amount of energy to maintain itself.

This is because the sphere has the least amount of surface area for a given volume.

This cohesion of water generates a tension on its surface. Surface tension can be measured, and is the amount of force that is required to break or tear the surface of water apart.

When this surface is unbroken, water can support o6jects that are heavier. This is why boats can float, and why certain insects can run on the surface of water as if it were a solid.

We can float a needle on the surface of water as long as we do 'break' the surface.

Not only is water attracted to itself, it is also attracted to solid substances. The degree of its adhesion depends on the substance in which it comes into contact.

This process of adhesion is called wetting. The ability of pure water to wet a substance is dependent on the electric charge of the water molecule and the nature of the substance.

Some substances such as paraffin cannot be 'wet' by water, whereas other substances such as glass, cotton, clays, and rocks are easily wet by water. In fact, nearly all inorganic and organic substances found in nature can be wet by water.

All substances have what is known as wetting index. This index is representative of the surface tension required to wet that substance. In the food processing industry it is well known that certain food substances cannot be wet by ordinary water. The thermodynamics of wetting is determined by the value of the contact angle between the solid particle and the water.

Contact angle is a function of surface tension. Any solid substance has its own critical surface tension, Y_c, which is required for wetting. Any liquid with a surface tension below Y_c will wet the solid. Y_c = 39 dynes/cm for wetting starch at 20° C. The value for cellulose is 45 dynes/cm, while skim milk powder can we wetted by ordinary 73 dyne/cm water.

As we shall see later, when water is heated its surface tension decreases. This is why hot water will easily mix with some substances that will not be wet at all by cold water.

We can see that the surface tension of water becomes an extremely important factor in the absorption and assimilation of food by the body. This is the reason it is not good to drink ordinary water when we eat. Our digestive juices have a relatively low surface tension and readily 'wet' our food. When we drink ordinary bulk water which has a surface tension of 73 dynes per centimeter it dilutes the digestive juices and prevents adequate wetting of food particles

CHAPTER 3

WATER IS A LIQUID CRYSTAL
WITH AN ELECTRIC CHARGE

As our readers will recall, a simple molecule of water is composed of two gases. It consists of two hydrogen atoms bound to an oxygen atom as shown in the diagram.

This particular configuration is a distribution of electrons which results in uneven distribution of electric charge in each molecule.

This type of molecule is called a polar molecule, as its charges are distributed asymmetrically to form positive and negative poles. These molecules may be likened to an odd shaped battery.

The hydrogen and oxygen atoms of simple water molecules are so tightly bound that it takes a great deal of energy to separate or dissociate them into their free gaseous states.

Pure water contains only a tiny percent of pure hydrogen (H^+) and hydroxide (DH7) ions in free form.

Chapter 3

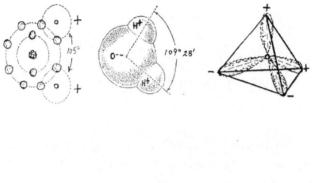

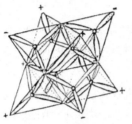
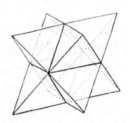

WATER MOLECULES

The basic water molecule is made of two hydrogen atoms and one oxygen atom as shown above. The bond angle between the two hydrogen atoms' nuclei is 104.5°. Some molecules are energized and have an angle of 109.5°. These energized molecules form the basis of the 'liquid crystal.' The electron orbital energy diagram of the water molecule forms a tetrahedron. The most stable liquid crystal is formed from eight of these tetrahydronal molecules. This form is called the Stella Octangula after Kepler.

This means that pure water is a very poor conductor of electricity since conductivity of liquids is dependent upon the existence of free ions. The high polar charge of the water molecule gives it as strong tendency to orient itself in an electric field.

The degree of orientation to an electric field is called the dipole moment. The size of the dipole moment is dependent on the physical charge separation within the molecule. Water has an unusally large dipole moment.

It is this dipole moment of the molecule that gives water some of its anomalous characteristics. When an electric field is applied to pure water, the alignment of molecules tends to neutralize the field. This ability of a substance to neutralize an applied electric field is called the dielectric constant of the material.

The dielectric constant of a vacuum is said to be 1. The dielectric constant of water is 80.

This means that two free electronic charges of same value in water will repel each other only 1/80th as much as the same charges would in a vacuum. It is water's dipole moment that enables it to dissolve substances.

These substances are held together by ionic bonds. Ionic bonded substances are held together by Coulombic Force, which is the attraction of one electric charge for another. These bonds are relatively weak when compared to other types of bonds.

For example, ordinary table salt with a formula of NaCl consists of an atom of sodium bound to an atom of chlorine. When salt is dry, the ions are bound to each other. When salt is placed in water, however, these weak bonds are broken and the molecules dissociate into Na* and Cl ions that have positive and negative charges.

These ions then move around in the water by thermal agitation but cannot recombine into salt because the dielectric constant of water is such that the attraction is 1/80th what it would be in a vacuum. (Note: the dielectric constant of air is very close to that of a vacuum).

The reason water molecules have such a high dipole moment is because the molecules attach to each other in such a way that the charges add up in the same way we get higher voltages by adding batteries in series.

The force that enables water molecules to form long chains of complex structures is known as the hydrogen bond. Going back to the basic water molecule, we can see that positively charged nuclei of the hydrogen atoms are exposed because the electrons are circulating in the electron orbits of the oxygen atom.

This produces a powerful positive electrostatic force which is known as the hydrogen bond.

If the water molecules are highly structured, the power of the hydrogen bond is increased because of the additive charges. It is the power of the hydrogen bond that enables water to wet substances such as glass, cotton, etc.

The positive hydrogen and the negative oxygen charges bind to electric charges present on the surface of the substance into which the water comes into contact.

The reason water does not wet paraffin is because paraffin is a non-polar molecule, and has no electric charge sites for the hydrogen bonds to act.

When water begins to freeze, the hydrogen bonds begin to form liquid crystal structures. The basic form of these structures is hexagonal.

When ice finally forms, it is composed of tetrahedrons that form larger hexagonal structures as seen in snowflakes.

Ordinary water, however, is not pure H_2O. It has a highly complex structure which is composed of random molecules of ordinary water which frantically move around by thermal agitation. Each molecule has an energy field which is called the electron orbital. In the singular water molecule, this orbital forms a tetrahedron with two positive charges and two negative charges on the vertices of the tetrahedron.

Within this sea of chaos float liquid crystal structures of water molecules that are highly organized. These liquid crystals consist of water molecules that are joined together.

These molecules are bound to one another by the hydrogen bond. This was predicted in the classical work of J. Bernal and R. Fowler, and was confirmed by X-ray diffraction studies. Tetrahedrons can be joined together in a certain number of limited ways. These molecular icebergs are made of clumps of tetrahedrons which are stable only in certain configurations. This may be represented by the following: Whereas the single molecule may be represented as H_2O, the iceberg may be represented as $(H_2O)_n$, where n= 1, 2, 3, 4, etc. The perfect water 'crystal' will have a number of 8. When tetrahedrons are joined together in an eight configuration the structure forms the Stella Octangula, a figure originally discovered and named by Kepler. This structure would be extremely stable.

Intermixed with these multiple tetrahedral crystal structures are free water molecules which are not bound by hydrogen bonds. This is the 'sea of chaos.' These molecules partially fill the loose packing regions within the water, structure.

Water in the living system is highly structured, that is, it is composed of a high percentage of Octangula liquid crystals with a very low percentage of chaotic unorganized molecules. Bulk water, on the other hand, is composed of a large number of random molecules which contain a small number of structured liquid crystals. There is a constant heat exchange process between structured tetrahedral molecules, and those which are not hydrogen bonded or structured. This is the result of thermal motion.

When an animal or plant takes in ordinary bulk water it has to create organized liquid crystals before the water can play a role as a vital living fluid.

This structuring is accomplished by means of high energy colloids. High energy means colloids that have a high electric charge. The living systems manufacture these colloids from minerals, albumins, albuminoids and polysaccharides (sugar complexes).

These colloids act as tiny 'seeds' of energy charge which attract water molecules and thus form the nucleus of a liquid crystal.

Colloids can only act as seed crystal nuclei it they have a high electrical potential. The charge on ordinary colloids is not very stable. In nature we see three different types of colloids.

The first is called an unprotected colloid. This is the kind of particle found in ancient sea beds. It is a type of clay. The surface of the colloid is exposed to agents that may discharge it. This colloid's particles remain discrete by mutual electrical repulsion. This repulsion is known as the Coulomb Force. Because its surfaces are bare, it is easily discharged by contaminants of the opposite charge. Clays all have a negative charge which is usually quite small.

The second colloid is found in living systems and is protected by a lyophilic (blending well with water) coating such as gelatin, albumin, or collagen. This coating protects the colloid from discharge because the coating's affinity for water exceeds the mutual attraction of adjacent particles.

The third type of colloid has a protective coating which is composed of a non-ionic (neutral change) polymer. The polymer must have a molecular chain length of around 10 to 12 carbon atoms to be effective. These coatings act as insulators and keep the colloids far enough apart to prevent them from discharging and joining or coagulating. When these colloids approach each other the osmotic pressure builds up between them. This pressure causes the solvent fluid (water) to rush in between and drive the particles apart. This type of colloid is found extensively in living systems and is the most stable colloid. This type of protection is used in most living fluids. This is the type of colloid which is found in Hunza and Crystal Energy.

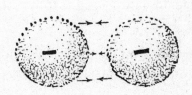

First Type of Colloid
Unprotected colloids repel each
other by electrostatic charge

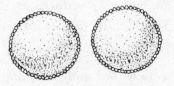

Second and Third Types
Protected colloids found in
living systems. Two types of
coatings are found - albuminoid
and oil

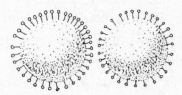

Fourth Type
Protected by a polar molecule of
soap. Used industrially and in
detergents not found naturally
in the living system

Four Types of Colloids

Concentrate™ water. It is rarely found outside the living system. In Hunza water this polymer coating apparently comes from a very fine organic oil that is found in some plants. It may also be found in some types of petrified wood.

There is a fourth type of colloid which is not found naturally in the living system, but is manufactured industrially and used as a detergent. This colloid is protected by ionic surfactants such as sulfated castor oil. These colloids are protected by a coating of ionic detergent. Such detergent molecules are polar. They have at one end a lyophilic molecule, and at the other end a lipophilic (likes oil) molecule. These are then attached to the colloid in such a way that the lipophilic side is on the inside facing the colloid, and the lyophilic end is facing into the fluid of suspension.

CHAPTER 4

NOVALIS FRAGMENTE
THE SENSITIVE CHAOS

Water is extremely sensitive to external energy forces. Dr. Theodore Schwenk of Weleda laboratories has written a very interesting book entitled *Sensitive Chaos*.

In his book he details water's great sensitivities to internal and external forces. Our relationship to water has drastically changed in the last few centuries.

Water is so commonplace we tend to take it for granted. In the past, fetching water was one of mankind's primary tasks. It involved. great effort and labor, men believed that water was inhabited by divine beings whom they could only approach with great reverence.

Like fire, air and Earth, water was one of the great spiritual beings that made up the whole of our world. With the beginning of the technological age of science, all but a few people lost their perception of the true nature of water.

Water is the bearer of the formative living process. The fluid element is the universal element, not yet solid but remaining open to outside influences, the unformed, indeterminate element, ready to receive definite form, they knew it as the "sensitive chaos" (Novalis, *Fragments*).

As man learned to use water technically and became familiar with its nature, the more his knowledge of the soul and spirit of this element faded.

Man no longer looked at the spiritual being of water, but only at its value in commerce. Today he has polluted the entire water element of the Earth, the very source and mother of life.

The destruction of the elements of Earth is fed by a way of thinking that perceive personal profit above the vital coherence of all things in nature.

Humanity has not only lost touch with the spiritual nature of water, but is in danger of losing its very physical substance. In the not so distant future, pure water will be more valuable than oil or gasoline.

All flowing water, though it may appear to be uniform is divided into extensive inner surfaces. In flowing streams, millions of vortexes form when water breaks past stones, sticks, and other obstructions. These vortex patterns act as powerful resonant structures as well as energizers and electrifiers for water and colloids.

These vortex flows are one of the secrets of water's great sensitivity to the forces of the universe.

Close observation reveals that the vortex has a rhythm of its own, it extends and contracts in a rhythmic pulsation. The vortex is really composed of a series of discrete flowing surfaces all bound together as if by an invisible hand.

These flowing interfaces move at different speeds, slow on the outside and fast on the inside.

The velocity of movement of water in a vortex multiplied by the radius from the center is a constant. This means that the velocity at the center of a vortex is theoretically infinite. As the forces in a perfect vortex approach infinity the bonds of the water molecule cannot sustain the pressure and begin to dissociate releasing powerful forces.

Water is sensitive to magnetic, electric, gravitational and vibratory influences. It is affected by light, sound and pressure. All these sensitivities are fleeting.

That is why magnetic treatment of water is ineffective. The only time water is really sensitive to external forces is when it is flowing.

When water flows, millions molecular. interfaces open up along interior flow lines. These interfaces are stretched like rubber bands and are so sensitive that they can be impressed by the subtle energies of planetary relationships.

In one experiment which was duplicated by Dr. Schwenk, Dr. Kolisko was able to show repeatable changes in crystallization of various mineral salts which were affected by planetary transits.

These energies are captured in water that is undergoing turbulent or vortical flow. The moment the flow is ceased, the energy of the moment is retained in the water until it is agitated or moved again, at which point a whole new set of energies are captured.

A lot has been written about magnetic and electrostatic treatment of water to prevent boiler scale and to enhance the growth of plants.

As we can see from the work of Schwenk, the effects of magnetic and electric fields on the structure of water are fleeting.

CHAPTER 5

MAGNETIC AND PSYCHIC
TREATMENT OF WATER

Patrovsky Venceslav of Czechoslovakia ran a number of tests on magnetically treated water to see what might be the cause of the positive effects attributed to magnetically treated or psychically energized water. (Influence of Some Force Fields including the Psi Field on Water).

In the case of the water treated by psychic energy, the water was energized by means of laying on of hands (hand passes over a container of water) or had been gazed upon for a period of time.

He found that treated water contained a small percentage of hydrogen peroxide or H_2O_2.

Hydrogen peroxide is formed out of ordinary water when its molecules are dissociated by an energy force.

In nature, this is formed by the act of cosmic rays or ultraviolet light acting on the surface of water.

An example of the formation of hydrogen peroxide in water can be seen when we add small fish to distilled water. These fish rapidly die because the water is free of dissolved oxygen.

If the water is poured back and forth a few times to dissolve atmospheric oxygen and fish are then added to the water a larger percentage live.

However, when distilled water is placed in sunlight for a while the ultraviolet light stimulates the production of hydrogen peroxide which is a powerful source of free oxygen. When fish are added to sunlight stimulated water the fish thrive.

By using a reagent made up of hemoglobin and a powerful fluorescent dye, Venceslav was able to detect hydrogen peroxide in extremely small quantities.

When these reagents are mixed with water that contains small quantities of peroxide, the water glows in the dark as the oxygen from the peroxide combines with the hemoglobin molecules.

As a result of this experiment, he was able to determine that water molecules can not only be dissociated by means of magnets, but also by the subtle energies which are emitted from the human hand and eyes.

The content of hydrogen peroxide was small, on the order of a few parts per million.

When energized, water was given to small seeds, the seeds germinated faster and in greater number than the control seeds.

The seeds given treated water also grew larger and healthier plants. As a final test to see if there was perhaps some ingredient in treated water that he had missed, he then tested magnetically energized water against water to which he had added a small amount of hydrogen peroxide.

The test results came out the same: the plants which were fed magnetically energized water and peroxide-treated water were identical.

Although these experiments tend to answer many of the questions regarding the healing effects of 'activated' water, they do not explain how magnetically treated water would deposit less scale on steam boilers.

Magnetically treated water has been used since the turn of the century for corrosion control, and as yet no one has really come up with a satisfactory explanation for this phenomenon.

CHAPTER 6

CRYSTAL TREATED WATER

In 1974, I purchased a Fisher Model 21 DuNuoys Ring Surface Tensiometer.

This device measures the surface tension of a fluid by means of a calibrated platinum wire ring.

It measures the cohesive force of water by placing the platinum ring in contact with a sample of water. The water sample wets the ring and adheres to the wire surface.

When a switch is thrown, an electric motor begins to rotate a calibrate torsion wire balance in an effort to lift the wire from the water surface.

As tension is increased on the torsion wire, the water surface begins to distort as the ring is lifted higher and higher. At a certain point, the water surface will rupture and the wire ring will break free from the surface.

At that point, the motor is automatically turned off, and the force required to lift the ring from the surface can be read on a calibrated dial.

This force is calibrated in dynes per centimeter, a unit of force. Ordinary water at room temperature has a surface tension of about 73 dynes per centimeter.

If we add energy to the water sample by means of heat, the cohesive force or surface tension is decreased.

As we heat water from room temperature to boiling the surface tension will be reduced from 73 dynes to 60 dynes.

One of the reasons that hot water is so effective in making coffee or tea, and in cleaning dirt from clothes is because of this reduction in surface tension.

The increased energy and reduced surface tension of water means that water will wet these substances easier. It also means that the water will penetrate through small openings with less force.

In our research into anomalous water behavior, we tried measuring all kinds of physical parameters and found that surface tension was an excellent measure of free energy contained in the water molecule.

If we lower the surface tension of water while maintaining temperature at a constant we can calculate the increase in free energy content of the water.

For example, if we lower the surface tension of room temperature water from 73 to 60 dynes/cm we have reduced the surface tension to the same level as that of boiling water.

In August of 1974, I found that crystals of all types had an effect on the surface tension, and therefore the structure of water

As an experiment we took a quartz crystal carefully cleaned with an ether solvent to ensure that it does not have anything such as oils or other surfaces active agents on its surface. We then lower the quartz crystal into a 100 millimeter petri dish containing 50 millimeters of distilled water.

Prior to adding the crystal we measure the surface tension of the distilled water and find it to be 73 dynes/cm. After adding the crystal to the water we wait a few minutes and gently remove the crystal from the dish.

Without agitating the water we then measure surface tension again and find that it has lowered. Typical reductions of 10 dynes per centimeter are common.

If we vigorously agitate the water or stimulate the surface by means of an arc from a Tesla Coil high voltage generator (electrical agitation) the water will lose its free energy and the surface tension will go back up to 73.

If we had added a chemical surfactant to the water, agitation would not increase the surface tension. We were somehow increasing the energy of the fluid by means of the crystal. We were changing the structure by an energy effect.

In order for an energy change to occur, there must be an energy source. Crystals are excellent receptors of all kinds of energy from the cosmos. Remember our crystal radios?

We wondered if the crystal effect might be the missing factor that affects Hunza water. We speculated that the ground in Hunzaland was filled with quartz crystals, and that the energy of the crystals was somehow transferred to the water.

Kings of old used to drink their water and wine out of jeweled goblets made of gold. Other members of the court drank their beverages from goblets made of crystals and pure zinc.

One way to test the life-giving qualities of water is to test its effects on plants. We found that the crystal effect would persist as long as the water was not disturbed in a turbulent way. When crystal treated water was poured it had to be done so in a laminar fashion.

For test plants we chose a number of seeds such as wheat, mung bean, soy, alfalfa and radish. In all our tests, the activated water produced a more vigorous growth. The sprouts produced by this water were sweeter, larger and more. delicious.

We filled brandy snifters with precious and semi-precious crystals such as rubies, diamonds and quartz. Every evening before going to bed we would fill our snifters with distilled water to be treated overnight.

In the morning we would carefully drink the activated water creating as little turbulence as possible. tale could definitely feel the energy effect of the crystal activated water. It acted as a powerful diuretic and increased our energy. I spent hours designing machines that would treat water with crystals.

There was only one problem. The problem of turbulence. When we take crystal energized water into the stomach it undergoes terrific agitation before it reaches the bloodstream. Once in the blood it undergoes more agitation, Also, the water in Hunzaland was taken from a turbulent stream that originated from a melting glacier.

Crystals could not be the answer if the water was tumbled to the point where any semblance of structure would be destroyed. Crystal energized water cannot be stored or shipped due to the ephemeral nature of this phenomenon.

CHAPTER 7

WE TEST HUNZA WATER

At this point in our research, Betty Lee Morales, who had enthusiastically expressed support for our work, returned from a trip to Hunzaland with a sample of Hunza water for me to test.

On examination of the water sample we found that it was extremely cloudy. Betty told us that Hunza people believed the cloudy minerals in Hunza water were the source of thein good health. The answer lay in the cloudy minerals.

The surface tension of the Hunza sample was 68 dynes per centimeter. If the water was vigorously shaken, the tension would go up to 72 or so, and on remaining still for a few moments would return to 68. This indicated that a structuring was taking place.

I wondered if the cloudy minerals were tiny crystals that altered the water like our larger quartz crystals.

We sent the water to have it analyzed. When the analysis of the Hunza sample was returned we found that the cloudy minerals were colloidal silicates. The cloudy minerals were not crystals but amorphous silica minerals that had a high zeta potential or electric surface charge. These minerals would be harmless to take internally as they were soft and had no sharp edges. They were a type of clay particle colloid that was protected by a thin coating of nonionic organic polymer. The reason why these colloids were so effective was because of this fine coating. It was a type of oil that would come from plants or from plants that had been petrified. Some types of petrified wood contain this type of oil.

We will delve into the properties of colloids later, but at this point we can say that colloids are tiny insoluble particles that have a negative electric charge.

These particles are so tiny that the normal thermal agitation of water keeps them suspended. The electric charges cause colloids to repel each other so that an electrical field pattern is created in the water in which they are suspended.

As living colloids have a negative electric charge, any substance that has a positive electric charge will destroy the charge on the colloids and cause them to agglomerate or flocculate. When this happens they fall out of suspension.

After years of research we had the answer. The negatively charged colloids in Hunza water act as small nuclei for liquid crystals. These highly charged hydrated particles structure the water in much the same way as fluids are structured by the living plant or animal system.

At this point I reasoned that the structuring of water by means of quartz crystals was also an electrical phenomenon.

To test my theory I took a quartz crystal and tested its effect on water. It reduced the surface tension from 73 to 55 dynes.

I then took the crystal and sprayed the entire surface with the brush discharge from a 100,000 volt Tesla coil. The 'brush' discharge is an electrical brush of ionized air that contains positive and negative electrical charge. The 'brush' acted as an electrical charge neutralizer. It effectively would erase any electrical charge from the surface of the crystal.

If my theory was right, the neutralized crystal would have no structured surface charge and would not affect the water at all.

After treating the crystal I placed it back in a petri dish of water and it had no effect on surface tension at all.

Did I permanently destroy the crystal? I tested the crystal every day and found that it slowly regained its charge and ability to alter water.

Where does this charge come from? Our tests indicate that monopolar gravity waves may charge the crystals. Quartz crystals are resonators for cosmic energy impulses.

As these waves fill the entire universe and are generated by novas, supernovas, and starquakes they are plentiful. We recently made a crystal gravity wave detector. This device consists of a quartz crystal with wire electrodes attached at each end. These wires are then fed into a low noise high gain amplifier. Any tiny voltages generated by the crystal are then amplified and fed into a chart recorder. The entire apparatus is enclosed in a mu-metal box which shields it from ordinary electromagnetic waves. We have shown that this device does indeed pick up cosmic gravity waves. These are converted into electrical charges on the surface of the crystal.

Signals from the crystal are amplified by a sensitive amplifier and can be heard through a loudspeaker or displayed by means of an oscilloscope or chart recorder.

Perhaps colloids are also sensitive to gravity waves. The experiment discussed earlier which was performed by Dr's Schwenk and Kolisko tend to support this theory.

WE TRY TO DUPLICATE HUNZA WATER

Having realized that the crystal activation of water was due to the highly structured electric charges on the surface of crystals, and that the structure of Hunza water was due to the electrical charge on protected high energy colloids, we tried to duplicate Hunza water by adding different colloidal clays to distilled water.

We tested clays from an ancient sea bed in Utah, and numerous clays from all over the world. None of the clays tested worked. The problem was that these colloids did not have a high electrical charge and the particles were too large to be used by the living system. The charge on clays is very low, in the range of a few millivolts only.

The electrical change on the colloids from Hunzaland is around 40 millivolts (0.040 volts). This may not seem like much, but add 1,000,000 of these particles to a glass of water and the total charge would be 0.040 X 1,000,000 = 40,000 volts!

The electric charge on colloids is called zeta potential or ZP for short. The zeta potential on all colloids in living systems is negative or minus.

Our next step was to attempt creation of these high zeta potential Hunza colloids in our laboratory. I worked on hundreds of formulas over a period of five years and did not succeed in creating colloids that acted like the ones from Hunzaland.

CHAPTER 8

THE ALCHEMICAL DREAM
HUNZA WATER IS DUPLICATED

In August of 1982 Gael and I met for the first time at a seminar in Phoenix, Arizona. Gael was known as the Crystal Lady since she had been involved in crystal research for over 15 years. She has one of the most beautiful natural crystal collections I have ever seen. After the seminar she went to live in the forest in a house full of crystals. She lived there for a year while continuing her crystal research.

We met again in August, 1983 when we were both lecturing at another seminar in Scotsdale, Arizona. This meeting was definitely our destiny; as an inner knowing exploded into consciousness we knew that we were twin flames (souls) and that we would be together for the rest of our lives.

We have never been apart since that second meeting. We moved to a remote ranch in northern Arizona where we established a research laboratory. Shortly after moving into our new home we had an overwhelming desire to go to Egypt and spend the night in the Great Pyramid of Giza. We also found that Gael's friend Beverly Criswell another crystal person was, also planning on going to Egypt.

On November 14th we met at the Mana House Oberoi. This elegant hotel was built by Napoleon Bonaparte as a palace for Josephine. Our goal was to get our small group into the King's Chamber of the Great Pyramid on the evening of November l8th. This particular evening was the peak of a three day Pleiadian star alignment that Beverly said only occurs every 4,800 years. This was to be a very special time in history and we wanted to be the ones inside the Great Pyramid on this auspicious occasion.

It is virtually impossible to get permission to stay all night in the Great Pyramid. It is locked up every evening at 6:00 p.m. and' the key is stored in plain sight on the wall of the police station in Giza. You can not even bribe your way in, permission must be given. Fortunately, fate was with us as we obtained permission to stay in the pyramid for the entire night.

At 4:00 in the afternoon on the 17th Gael and I made the long climb inside the pyramid to the King's Chamber level. We were both dressed in white. Once in the chamber, a minister friend of ours whom we brought to Egypt for this purpose performed a special 'soul mate' ceremony in front of the King's' coffer. We were the first couple in history to be married in the Great Pyramid.

At 11:00 p.m. on November 18th, we entered the King's Chamber with a very small group of crystal 'initiates.' On the evening of November 11th, on the Full Moon, Gael and I climbed the equivalent of fifty stories to the top of the pyramid where we spent the night alone in meditation. She also placed special quartz crystals in secret places on the apex. Our night in the pyramid will be the subject of yet another book.

After spending another two weeks visiting the sacred places and temples of ancient Egypt we flew to Greece where we spent our honeymoon visiting the sacred temples of this ancient country.

We then returned home to our retreat in northern Arizona.

Shortly thereafter we were inspired to begin a liquid fast.

On the 22nd fasting day we were taking our daily six mile walk when our conversation turned to the supreme importance of water and high energy colloids. When we returned home we went into the laboratory and began a new series of experiments.

We created a special device which can only.be described as a Vortex Tangential amplifier. This apparatus creates a perfect liquid vortex. As the newly formed colloids are fed into the vortex they are subjected to forces which cannot be created any other way.

Nature generates these forces every day. We have such vortex amplifiers in the living body. As the colloids were fed into the vortex, they were enhanced even further by means of an electronic energy field. This field is applied at precisely the correct moment, when the center, or eye of the vortex, is less than one millionth of an inch in diameter.

The colloids we created changed the surface tension of distilled water from 73 dynes per centimeter to an all-time low of 25 dynes! When we measured the zeta potential or electric charge of these new colloids it was a record high. The charge was 125 millivolts. If we add 1,000,000 of these particles to a glass of water, the total change would be 1,000,000 X 0.125 = 125,000 volts.

At this point we decided to continue our fast on our new high energy Hunza water colloids. At the end of 40 days we decided to switch from orange juice and Hunza water to a liquidarian diet.

The liquidarian diet was essentially a whole juice diet. The daily drinks were made by first putting a quart of our new colloidal activated water in a blender.

We then added various fruits or vegetables depending on how we felt. Gael then added a special spice mix which she named Herbal Enlightenment.

The drinks were so delicious we seldom if ever missed eating. Our liquidarian diet continued for six months. During that period we ate no solid foods, only liquefied foods which were always fortified with our Hunza colloids. We maintained perfect health and body weight during the entire fast. We both felt wonderfully clear and light.

This was in August, 1984. Everyone who saw us said that we looked better and healthier than ever. They said that our eyes had a wonderful clarity and were as bright as headlights. They all wanted some of our water. Before long we were distributing our water to about 2,000 people and had changed the name from Hunza water: to Crystal Energy Water™.

In October we went to Florida and were married again at the Unity Center which is said to be the site of an old Atlantean temple. A double rainbow appeared over the top of the church right after our ceremony. The Unity wedding was our legal wedding in the United States. It was also a celebration of the birth of our new Crystal Energy Water™.

When we returned to Arizona we went into seclusion to continue our research in order to further perfect our colloids. Over the next year, we were able to perfect our colloids far beyond those from Hunzaland.

Experimentally we found that the ideal surface tension to eliminate stored toxins was between 55 and 65.

Our Crystal Energy Concentrate colloids are adjusted so that when they are diluted for drinking the surface tension was in the above range.

CHAPTER 9

THE IMPORTANCE OF COLLOIDS
IN THE LIVING SYSTEM

"In fact today colloids may be regarded as important, perhaps the most important connecting link between the organic and inorganic world."

Wolfgang Pauli

The medium in which life is found is known as the colloidal medium. We know today, that all living organisms are composed, of highly structured colloids or liquid crystals, and that these form the basis of a gigantic colloidal computer.

Colloidal science is young and little is known about. these high-energy molecules. Science has accumulated a wealth of data on colloids but has not as yet developed a general theory about their behavior. Most of the work on colloids has been in the use of colloids in industrial processes. Little is known about colloids in the living system.

Recent discoveries by Dr. Fritz Albert Popp from Germany indicate that the DNA molecule transmits its blue-print information to other cells by means of an encoded burst of coherent ultra-violet laser light.

The optical pathway that transmits this information consists of highly structured cellular water. (Fusion Magazine, Sept-Oct 1985) The structure of cellular water is determined by minute quantities of highly charged colloidal minerals.

To gain a working conception of what colloidal chemistry is, consider that living tissues and organs are simply great masses of cells—billions of them. The energy, the very life-force of these cells, is obtained from certain minerals and metals, among them iron, iodine, manganese and copper. There are some 32, with traces of as many others, in the human body. Colloidal chemistry is the science which converts those elements into particles so minute that they can be utilized by living cells.

The effect of colloids is explainable in part by electric action' Sick and dead and broken down cells are attracted to the colloids by electro-magnetic force, as iron filings are attracted to a magnet. The colloids carry those decayed or poisonous substances into the bloodstream, and they are eliminated, the system meanwhile adapting what it needs of the colloids.

A simple illustration will suggest the immense powers that are being unsealed.

Suppose we have a cube of iron measuring an inch on each edge. The total surface would be six square inches. The electrical charge is on the surface; therefore, the greater the surface the greater the charge; and if we divide the cube of iron into smaller pieces we increase the surface areas. By colloidal chemistry, that iron cube can be divided into particles so minute that they are invisible, hence instead of six square inches of surface emanating electric energy, we have something like 127 acres.

(See Reader's Digest, March 1936)

The smallest particle that can be seen by a microscope is 1,000 times as large as a molecule.

These small particles are known as the "Twilight Zone of Matter."

(See: Korzybski: *Science and Sanity*)

In this fine range of subdivided matter we find the peculiar forms of behavior known as 'colloidal behavior.'

As we divide matter into smaller and smaller particles, the surface area of the particles increases at a geometric rate. Colloidal particles have such a large surface area that a quarter of a teaspoon of particles has a surface area greater than that of a football field.

Because of this great surface area, colloids generate surface energies that have powerful effects on physical and chemical reactions. (Gustave LeBon: *Evolution of Energy*)

Certain colloids act as powerful catalysts in chemical reactions often behaving like enzymes in life processes. Because of their small size and large surface energies, the, electrical characteristics of colloids become of fundamental importance as all surfaces are made up of electrical charges.

Electrical charges have the well-known property that like charges repel, and opposite charges attract. The combination of high surface energies and electrical charges that may accompany colloids accounts for the action and sensitivity of colloids in the living system.

The higher the electrical potential on the surface of a colloid, the more active it is as an energy source. The electrical charge on the surface of a colloid is known as the 'zeta potential.'

CHAPTER 10

ELECTRICITY 1N THE BLOOD

Science, religion and philosophy are in complete agreement on one and only one subject—the quality and the power of life is dependent on the blood.

The ancient Chinese named the circulatory system the 'Red Dragon,' There are special secret exercises known as the Red Dragon System. These exercises are said to energize and charge the blood with CHI or life energy. They are performed with a wooden rod two Chinese cubits in length.

The rod is held in different ways while a series of complex postures are performed which are meant to circulate this life energy to various parts of the body.

It is true that the blood system is the very key to health and longevity. Its proper function is necessary for feeding. every cell its proper nutrition, and for the elimination of cellular waste by-product as well as for defending the body against poisons, bacteria and disease viruses. Alexis Carrel received the Nobel prize in medicine for proving that the living cell is immortal if it is fed the proper nutrients and all toxic waste is removed.

The blood naturally does these things in conjunction with all the organs in the body. If the blood is in a state of imbalance the organ systems cannot do their jobs. The blood of animals is composed entirely of colloidal particles.

These colloids are bathed in a special electrolyte or ionic fluid that help keep the negative charge or zeta potential within a specific range.

Various types of stress in the form of ionic imbalances, certain electromagnetic waves, hormone imbalances or toxins and free radicals in the form of positive ions tend to destroy the negative on these living colloids.

When the negative potentials are reduced, the cells begin to agglomerate or gel in different degrees. The blood viscosity increases, the cells lose their discreteness and they cannot transport nutrients into cells and remove toxins from the body.

When these conditions persist oven a long period of time, the various body systems begin to function poorly. The body dies by degrees, inch by inch. What is known as disease is simply the body's response to the degradation of its efficiency by these things that destroy its electric charge.

Thomas Riddick, a pioneer colloid chemist, says that zeta potential is a basic law of nature. It plays a vital role in plant and animal life, and is the force that maintains the discreteness of the billions of circulating cells which nourish the organism. (Control of Colloid Stability through zeta potential).)

According to Riddick, colloidal particles are particles of matter that range in size from 100 Angstroms to 10 microns. Most organic colloids are in the 0.2 to 10 microns range in size.

Since these particles have a unipolar electric charge, they tend to be very stable in a solution of distilled water.

When electrolytes which are composed of positive and negative ions are added to the solution, the electrical charge on the colloids is altered by what is known as the double electric layer.

The electric double layer is formed in the following manner:

In distilled water, there are no free ions, so the colloids exist as discrete particles manifesting their individual charges, which are negative.

If a small amount of sodium chloride or salt is added to the system, the salt disassociates into individual sodium and chlorine ions. These ions each have a charge of one unit.

That is the sodium or Na^+ ions are positive and the chlorine, Cl^- ions are negative by one unit of charge.

Up to a certain concentration of ions, the sodium chloride ions will increase the zeta potential of the colloid in the following manner:

The Na^+ ions, which are called cations, will coat the colloid surface by a process of adsorption because opposite charges attract.

This coating of positive ions will form a rigid layer around the particle which is known as the Stern layer. The positive sodium ions form a layer on the surface of the colloid. This positive layer will then attract Cl^- ions to its surface.

The negative charges or anions will then form another diffuse layer around the Stern layer. These layers are like the layers of an onion.

The diffuse layer will merge into the bulk of the solution, which will contain a balanced quantity of positive and negative charges. This double layer will create a more. stable colloid and will also slightly increase zeta potential.

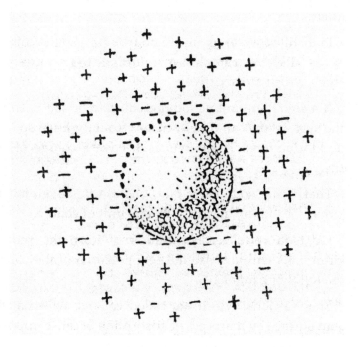

Colloidal Particle Double Layer

A negatively charged colloid tends to form a double layer of ions around its perimeter. The double layer acts to isolate and stabilize the electric charge on the surface of the colloid. The first layer is called the Stern layer and has a positive charge. It is surrounded by a diffuse layer of charges that extend into the bulk electrolytic solution. If too many free ions are found in the bulk, electric stress will become too great and the double layer will be destroyed. If a protective coating such as albumin is adsorbed onto the surface of the colloid, it will help to isolate the colloid's electric charge from ionic stress. Such a colloid will remain stable even in high ionic concentrations

The addition of specific electrolytes will increase zeta potential of the colloid up to a point. That point is when too much salt is added to the solution.

As more and more salt is added, the double layer will become thinner due to ionic electrical stress that is impressed on the particles.

At a certain point, the double layer will be ruptured and the colloid will discharge its voltage, resulting in a coagulation of the particles. They will all come together because they are no longer being repelled from each other by their like electrical charges.

If this were to happen in the human blood system, massive coagulation would occur throughout the body. This condition does happen, and when it does the person dies.

Mother nature stabilizes organic colloids by coating them with special polymers that effectively insulate the particle from loss of its electrical charge. Some of the more common polymers used in plants and animals are albumin, albuminoids and polysaccharides (sugar-like molecules). These coatings in combination with special polyelectrolytes form multiple protective layers around the colloid.

If an electrolyte such as potassium citrate is added to protected colloid the zeta potential is increased even further due to the fact that the citrate anion or negative ion has a charge of -3 while potassium has a charge of +1.

When colloids are suspended in a fluid such as water, they form a cloud like suspension of particles that tend to defy gravity.

Although these particles are heavier than water, the electrical potentials of the colloids keeps them in suspension.

This repulsion of particles creates a constantly moving particle plasma whose energy is far from equilibrium. The surface energies of the colloids tend to cause attraction to each other, while the electric charges tend to repel the particles away from each other. So long as colloids retain their charge, they are alive.

But, since colloids are in a high-energy state, they are unstable complexes that undergo continuous transformations

These transformations can be induced by light, heat, electric fields, electromagnetic forces, gravitational forces, solar flares and other forms of energy.

If the colloidal system loses its electrical charge, the system loses its colloidal behavior—it is 'dead.' This applies to both organic and inorganic systems.

In a previous example, we discussed the increase in zeta potential by the addition of potassium citrate electrolyte to a colloidal system.

This is known as an anionic electrolyte as potassium has a +1 charge and. The citrate molecule (from citric acid) has a change of -3. This is called a 1:3 electrolyte. It is said that the citrate molecule is trivalent. This means that it has three excess electrons. Potassium on the other hand is monovalent positive, which means that it is missing one electron. It therefore takes three potassium atoms to balance the -3 charge on: one citrate molecule.

Sodium chloride or salt is known as a 1:1 electrolyte as sodium and chlorine being monovalent have +1 and -1 charges respectively.

A positive ion is called a cation because it is attracted to the cathode or negative electrode. For example, if we put platinum electrodes in a glass of water and connect a 12 volt battery to these electrodes, the cations or positive ions will be attracted to the negative pole or cathode, and the anions or negative ions will be attracted to the positive electrode or anode. So negative ions are called anions as they are attracted to the anode or positive pole.

On the other hand, there are cationic electrolytes that have high positive charges. For example, if aluminum chloride is added to a colloidal solution the AL or aluminum ions have a +3 charge, while the CI or chlorine ions have a -1 charge. Thus aluminum chloride is a 3:1 electrolyte.

Since aluminum, is trivalent positive it has a +3 charge. Aluminum ions will therefore a negative organic colloid system and cause coagulation. This is due to the tremendous electric stress it presents to the system.

Thus aluminum ions in sufficient quantity destroy colloid stability in living systems. This is why aluminum deodorants and antacids are bad for us in spite of the fact that we are told they are harmless.

Aluminum ions are used in water purification plants to coagulate pollutants such as human waste. Most purification systems add too much aluminum to the water and the resulting excess ions end up in tap water.

All municipal water systems add chemicals to the water to coagulate or flocculate organic materials. They then add other minerals (cationic in nature) to condition the water so it doesn't corrode the city pipes.

These minerals are added without knowledge as to their potential danger in the living system.

Since the blood is a delicately balanced colloidal system with a negative zeta potential, the cationic electrolytes in tap water tend to cause blood clumping and aggregation in people who drink tap water.

No wonder cardiovascular disease is the number one killer!

Electrolytes can therefore be classed as either cationic or anionic. They are further defined by valence or ionic charge in the following way:

Multivalent cationic electrolytes have ions that have such a high positive charge that they must be balanced by numerous smaller anions.

These electrolytes are classified as 4:1, 3:1 and 2:1 ratios. The numbers on the left side of the colon designate the value of the positive charged ions in the chemical formula for that electrolyte. The numbers to the right of the colon represent the negative ionic charge value of the anions in the compound. In the 3:1 electrolyte the cation or positive ion of the compound has a charge of +3.

The anion side of the molecule has a charge of -1. Therefore, in the chemical compound, electronic balance is achieved by combining three anions to balance the charge of one +3 cation. Aluminum Chloride is a cationic electrolyte. The chemical formula is $AlCl_3$. As we can see three chlorine ions are needed to balance one aluminum ion.

When this substance is dissolved in a colloid solution the +3 aluminum ion is devastating to the negative electrical charges on the colloids.

Anionic electrolytes are mineral salts that are combined in the opposite way, they have multivalent anions or negative charges that must be balanced by multiple cations.

They are classed as 1:2, 1:3, 1:4 electrolytes. The anion is always the number on The right side, and the cation is always the number on the left side of the colon. Neutral electrolytes are the 1:1 charges.

In a given colloidal system, 3:1 electrolytes are up to 3,000 times as potent as 2:1 electrolytes and 6,000 times as potent as 1:1 electrolytes.

Since cationic electrolytes tend to discharge or kill colloidal systems, they can have devastating effects on living circulatory systems.

The reason cationic electrolytes are so dangerous to colloid stability is that the highly charged positive ions are attracted to the negatively charged colloids.

These highly charged cations destroy the stability of negative zeta potential colloids on contact.

On the other hand, anionic electrolytes tend to protect colloids from destruction and actually increase the negative potential on the colloid.

Examples of anionic electrolytes are: potassium sulfate (1:2), sodium sulfate (1:2), sodium citrate (1:3), potassium citrate (1:3), sodium pyrophosphate (1:4) etc. There are hundreds of others.

The blood of healthy humans consists of formed elements or suspensoids and plasma proteins or colloids in an aqueous suspension.

Dissolved in this system are approximately ly9 grams per liter of mineral salts of which sodium chloride is the principle constituent.

The amount of 1:1 sodium chloride in blood would normally destroy the stability of ordinary high zeta colloids. Blood has a protective protein that surrounds the blood colloids and acts as a barrier to discharge of the zeta potential. This protective barrier is albumin.

Albumin is a high polymer protein and is also a colloid of much smaller particle size than red blood cells, platelets, etc.

The albumin .is adsorbed onto the colloids and also onto the walls of the vessels and arteries. The albumin in turn adsorbs negative ions or anions onto its surface.

Blood also has anionic electrolyte to increase its zeta potential. Some of the natural anionic electrolytes in blood are various phosphates and citrates.

In health, the formed elements of blood remain discrete. They do not adhere to each other or to the blood vessel and arterial walls. This is due to the adsorption of electronegative plasma proteins on the surface of all the formed elements, and on the vessel walls. This creates mutual repulsion.

If the stability of this system is disturbed, that is the charge on these colloidal elements is reduced, the efficiency of the entire system is in jeopardy. If the instability continues, various forms of illness will ensue.

Stability is affected by diet, intake of mineral salts, and various forms of stress such as electromagnetic fields from fluorescent lights, television sets, computers, etc.

The stability of the colloidal charge in the blood is determined by the type of colloids and electrolytes present in the system.

Vegetation also depends on discrete colloidal fluid systems for its integrity. In vegetables, fruits and plants, the most likely colloidal protective mechanism is a combination of albuminoids (albumin-like) and anionic electrolytes.

We have found that all living fluids are liquid crystals and have structure which is due to colloids of high zeta potential.

In tests of blood serum, urine, vegetable and fruit juices, the surface tension of fresh fluids was very low, ranging from 65 for average blood serum to 30 for fresh carrot juice.

The colloids of living fluids however have a short life upon removal from the living cell. This may be due to a self-protective mechanism of gelation or clotting. This protective system is meant to protect the body from fluid loss in case of injury.

For example, in the human or animal body an injury resulting in the loss of fluid triggers the release of prothrombin which is a powerful cationic electrolyte that results in the coagulation of the fluid (blood clot). In this process prothrombin is converted into thrombin. Plants have a similar mechanism.

Take for example carrot juice: Fresh carrots were juiced using a Champion juicer. The resulting pulpy fluid was then filtered by means of a vacuum filter.

This removed all non-colloidal solids which were larger than 5 microns. The result was a clean colloidal fluid having a surface tension of 30.

When the juice extract was heated above 120°F., the surface tension rose to 73. Heating denatures and destroys albumin or albuminoids.

When the raw unheated juice was left in the refrigerator overnight, the surface tension rose to 68.

If left for a longer period, all charges were lost and the resulting had a surface tension of 73.

The natural clotting mechanism of carrot juice takes longer than the mechanism for blood. At the end of a given period of time the carrot juice was congealed or clotted in the bottom of the bottle.

Part of the clotting mechanism of juices may be attributed to microbial action as many microbes destroy the zeta potential of colloidal systems. This is probably due to the release of cationic substances as microbial waste products.

In our laboratories we have studied the surface tension of dozens of plant and vegetables juices. The juice with the lowest surface tension was carrot juice.

This juice is considered to have the greatest healing qualities of all juices. It is interesting to note that all food processing and cooking tends to destroy zeta potential in food.

These studies of highly charged colloids indicate that changed colloids in the living cellular fluid may be as important to our diets as enzymes, vitamins, etc.

When high potential colloids are added to pure water, the large surface forces alter its energy content as previously stated.

This is reflected by a change in the structure, of the water. Since water is in itself a liquid crystal of variable bonding. This means that the structure of water can be increased by adding charged colloids to the water.

When the structure of water is changed due to increased energy, the surface tension is reduced. Since energy is added without changing its temperature, the only way the liquid can absorb the energy is by changing its bonding pattern in order to accommodate the increase.

If we increase the energy in water by adding heat, the structure expands to accommodate the increased energy and the surface tension is reduced. When we add charged colloids to water, the energy is of an electrical nature, and the temperature does not change.

The increased energy is however reflected by a reduction of surface tension.

In Crystal Energy Concentrate™ colloids we create high zeta polysilicate minerals and then protect these minerals with an insulating coating of an organic polyelectrolyte.

Our protective polymer is more stable than albumin, as a result our colloids are so well protected that they maintain their charge under the most severe conditions.

They may be microwaved, frozen, boiled, autoclaved, irradiated wi.th gamma rays and immersed' in a number of powerful cationic electrolytes without losing their electrical charge.

A way of measuring the electrical change on colloids is by means of a U-shaped glass tube. The tube is filled with the colloidal solution. Platinum electrodes are placed in the ends of the tube, and an electrical potential is applied to the electrodes.

This is a type of electrophoresis cell. The colloids will all migrate toward one of the poles. If the colloid has a negative charge, it will migrate to the positive electrode. If the colloid has a positive charge, it will travel to the negative pole.

If the colloid has no charge, it will not migrate at all, but will settle in the bottom of the tube. The rate of migration for a given, electrical charge is determined by the zeta potential of the colloid.

Using this simple technique, we have established a direct relationship between zeta potential, surface tension, and the structuring effect on water.

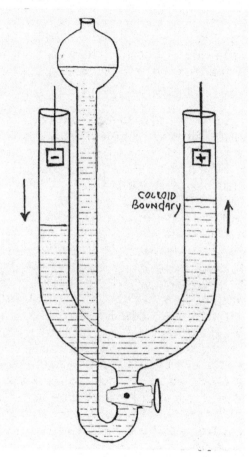

Electrophoresis Cell
for Measuring Zeta potential

The rate of migration of the colloidal boundary layer 1s a function of voltage applied and zeta potential. By measuring the rate of migration, zeta potential or colloidal charge can be calculated.

CHAPTER 11

THE COLLOIDAL COMPUTER

Although we have focused on blood as a high zeta potential biological-system, our bodies are composed entirely of colloids.

In fact, the human body is a nearly perfect colloidal computer. Every cell is made up of or is a colloid. These colloids are arranged to create specific functions.

Dr. Robert O. Becker of the Upstate New York Veteran's Hospital is considered to be the world's foremost authority on electrically accelerated healing of body tissues.

In his recent book *The Body Electric*, he describes his discovery of an analog computer healing system in the body. The nervous system is known as a digital information system. (This means information is transmitted by a series of pulses.) Becker has discovered that the cells surrounding the nerves, the glial cells in the brain, and the Schwann cells in the rest of the body form the basis of a direct current analog healing system.

In an analog computer, information is transmitted by voltage levels. When the body is injured, these cells set up a negative charge in the vicinity of the injury. This negative charge accelerates the healing process.

Many of our readers may recall that the difference between Einstein's brain and ordinary brains is that his brain had more glial cells. These cells surround the nerves and provide protection as well as nutritional substances.

Glial cells in the brain and Schwann cells in the rest of the body are made up of high zeta potential colloids which are arranged in a matrix.

Dr. Becker discovered that these cells are actually semiconductors just like transistors. He also discovered that there is a direct: correspondence between these cells and the acupuncture energy system!

The most highly structured water in the body is the water in the brain and nervous system. The water in the brain is so highly structured that it has been called 'ice' at 98.6' F (37"C). This structured water is also found in the cerebrospinal fluid. This fluid not only bathes the brain, but it extends down the entire length of the spine and extends through every nerve fiber from the top of the head to the tips of the toes. The distance covered by this liquid crystal is over 25,000 miles of nerve tissue. The human body is literally a gigantic liquid crystal!

The structure of biological liquid crystal water in the brain and nerves melts at about 106° F., this is interesting as that is also the body's core temperature at which people die.

The balance of electrolytes in the brain and nervous system is critical. The body has a special defense mechanism that prevents foreign substances from entering the brain. This is called the blood brain barrier.

It has been shown that the permeability of the blood brain barrier.is altered by external electric and magnetic fields of extremely low frequencies (ELF).

When unwanted materials enter this system the anionic electrolyte balance is disturbed and the crystalline structure of this vital liquid is changed.

Dr. Fritz Albert Popp of Germany has shown that our cells transmit DNA codes by ultraviolet laser light. He has shown that the mechanism of light transmission is by structured water molecules. He also indicates that these molecules of water are structured by colloidal minerals!

Since colloid pioneers such as Thomas Riddick believe zeta potential to be a basic law of nature, it becomes obvious that proper zeta potential is basic to life itself.

ELF signals are transmitted by hundreds of industrial and household products. Everything from hair driers, TV sets, computers, washing machines, clothes driers, even electric wrist watches emit these low frequency waves.

Dr. Becker believes the existence of the human race is threatened by these signals as they are altering the biochemistry of life itself.

Our experiments have shown that colloid stability is threatened by ELF signals when the zeta potential of the colloidal system is low. When colloids have a low zeta potential they are very unstable as the particles are on the verge of coagulation. At this point it takes very little stress to trigger gelation.

This occurs in most colloids at a zeta potential of around -10 millivolts (thousandths of a volt). Is it possible that by adding high energy zeta colloids and anionic electrolytes to the body, that the resulting increased zeta potential of the cells would protect us from these harmful energies?

CHAPTER 12

DIET AND COLLOIDS

As the purpose of this book is to discuss the discovery and use of liquid crystal water in the living system, the subject of diet though very important is secondary and will not be discussed here at great length. The only discussion of diet will be in regard to effects of diet on the integrity of the bio-colloidal system as it relates to zeta potential.

Since the colloids in the living system are complex structures whose zeta potential is protected by a coating of albumin or albuminoid substances which are then charged by anionic electrolytes, it would that the greatest cook of all our creator meant for us to eat a raw food diet. The ideal diet would be one which is high in juicy raw fruit, as fruit contains an abundance of high zeta potential colloids and anionic polyelectrolytes.

Any type of food processing such as cooking denatures the albuminoids and destroys zeta potential. It is well known that heat destroys enzyme activity but few realize that enzymes are high zeta potential colloids. Heat denatures the delicate protective coatings on the enzyme and destroys its charge. As a result, there is massive coagulation of fluids.

This destruction of colloidal discreteness makes the difference between 'live' and 'dead' foods.

Most nutritionists believe that enzymes make the difference between live and dead foods. It is becoming obvious that zeta potential may be the 'life energy' in enzymes.

As we mentioned in a previous chapter, we have tested the zeta potential and surface tension of blood serum, raw milk, urine and plant juices.

We have found that fresh raw fluids and juices from living organisms all have low surface tension and high zeta potential.

Any type of aging, or cooking of these fluids destroys the potential on the colloids resulting in coagulation and death to the colloid energy system.

The ideal diet would be one of raw fruits and vegetables with a few sprouted nuts and seeds.

In a period of three years Patrick went from a standard American diet to a 99% pure. fruitarian diet. He began by eliminating all animal products from his diet, this included all dairy products. As he became adjusted to vegetables and fruits, he gave up coffee, tea, and social drinking of any kind" At that point in time, his body was becoming so pure as a result of Crystal Energy Concentrate™ that it was able to tell him instantly what foods were good and what foods were bad for him. Our current diet consists of mostly raw fruits and vegetables with occasional seeds such as pumpkin, sunflower, and sesame.

Gael has been eating a diet of 99% uncooked fruits and vegetables for the last 18 years. She has maintained perfect health and has never had a cold in all that time.

During this process we discovered that refined (dead) food is a drug to most people. When they eat a particular food it acts as a stimulant to the nervous system. The stimulation creates a desire for another food that acts as a different stimulant which creates a new set of cravings. This process goes on ad infinitum.

The process of bodily purification releases the body from the above cravings and enables it to be free from this harmful cycle. The body then develops sensitivities that enable it to choose food that is ideally suited for it. This process cannot be forced. It is the result of a natural progression.

We are in the process of writing a book on own dietary observations in the future. The above information is for general interest only and is not meant to be a dietary recommendation for everyone. The real key to this puzzle is Liquid Crystal Water™, the elixir of the ageless.

Any discussion of diet is ancillary to the importance to the theme of this book. Coanda's words still ring true: "We are what we drink."

THINGS THAT DESTROY LIVING COLLOIDS

For the moment, we would like to discuss the various things in our lives that are 'bad' for us, these are those items that tend to reduce the zeta potential and therefore ruin the structure of our own delicate vital bodily fluids.

ALUMINUM

Aluminum is found everywhere in our lives. It makes a great building material but is deadly when taken into the human body.

The FDA considers aluminum to be harmless, but zeta potential studies show that it is far from the case. Instead of killing rapidly, it destroys slowly.

In colloidal systems, aluminum ions in the range of 4 parts per million cause total destruction of colloidal stability. Aluminum is used in some baking powders, antacids, deodorants, and soft drink cans.

Millions of people eat food and drink coffee that is made in aluminum cook ware and coffee pots. Campers often drink water that has been stored in aluminum canteens.

The first step toward optimum health would be to eliminate all aluminum from our food sources. Aluminum cans found in the multi-billion dollar soft drink and beer industry may leach aluminum ions into the beverage.

These cans have an inner liner that is supposed to keep this from happening, but the sealing process invariably causes damage to the liner and allows leaching to occur.

The only aluminum that is harmless is colloidal aluminum silicate contained in clays such as bentonite. These clays have a negative zeta potential.

There is sometimes.one problem however, when the clays are mined the people who process the clay first add anionic electrolytes such as sodium pyrophosphate to the clay to increase its zeta potential and liquid dispersion. This is so the clay can be handled easier.

The clay is then transported via pipelines to a processing plant where it is coagulated by the addition of aluminum cations. The clay is then washed, dried and packaged. The residue of 'the aluminum cations is then left in the clay.

Some of these clays are then sold to the health industry where bentonite intestinal cleansers are made.

Unprocessed clays in their natural state are powerful intestinal cleansers as they adsorb toxins from the intestinal walls and even pull toxins out of the blood stream as they pass through the intestinal canal.

Pure clays should have very little effect on the specific conductivity of distilled water. If electrolytes are added by processing, the electrolytes will affect the conductivity of distilled water when clay is added.

One way of testing for residual electrolytes is by adding a specific amount of clay to distilled water and, then testing for increase in specific conductivity with a special conductivity meter.

Our laboratory tests have shown that some of the clays sold in health food stores have been processed with cationic electrolytes.

PROCESSED FOODS

Thomas Riddick ran a test of mineral salt content of natural versus cooked foods. He found that the low sodium to high potassium content of natural foods is reversed by all food processors.

There is at present no federal limit on the amount of salt that can be used in food processing.

The only reason sodium salt is used in food processing is because it is cheap. In natural unprocessed foods, potassium exceeds sodium by a minimum of 5:1 and goes as high as 100:1. On the other hand in processed foods the ratio is reversed. The sodium can exceed potassium levels by as much as 1000:1.

Excessive sodium ions are more disruptive of zeta potential than are potassium ions. The reason for this is unknown.

The function of the kidneys is to maintain the electrolyte balance of the blood by elimination of salts that would destroy the zeta potential and therefore the discreteness of the blood system. They do this by selectively eliminating excess 1:1 and 2:1 cationic electrolytes. An excess of these minerals is disruptive to colloid stability.

Our kidneys try to hold on to anionic or negative electrolytes as these keep the zeta potential of bodily fluids at a high specific level.

Our kidneys are designed to handle between five and ten grams of mineral salts per day. The average American consumes 20 to 25 grams of salt on a daily basis.

Even if we do not salt our food, salt shows up in hidden ways put there by the food processing industry. As we grow older the function of our kidneys decreases reducing our ability to handle these excess salts.

As a result, salts back up in our bloodstreams and reduce the zeta potential of blood colloids. Over a period of time excess salts are stored in various parts of our bodies as the elimination system cannot handle them. The end result is obesity, high blood pressure, kidney and heart disease. The reason most people gain weight when they grow older is because of a lifetime of accumulated toxins.

Because most people eat processed foods they get very few anionic electrolytes in their diet. This anion deficiency causes the body to call on its deep reserves in an effort to keep the system in balance. This is however, a losing battle. Internal stress takes its toll by making various organ systems work at many times their normal capacity. Depletion of vital electrolytes and colloidal minerals eventually has a devastating effect on the entire system. As a result people die inch by inch not really knowing what is wrong.

WATER, WATER EVERYWHERE

A recent study of a major city's tap water shows that the main ingredient is water. The second, main ingredient is shredded toilet paper!

Most of the tap water in our cities is too thin to plow and too thick to drink. Municipalities treat sewage water by means of cationic electrolytes in an effort to precipitate and remove organic waste colloids so the water can be recycled as drinking water. Today's tap water is yesterday's toilet water.

Chemicals used to treat waste water are all positively charged electrolytes that are potentially destructive to colloid balance when ingested.

After organic colloids. are removed water is treated with other cationic electrolytes solely to protect the city pipes.

Drinking tap water is a slow form of suicide. We haven't even mentioned the 4,000 or so carcinogens that have been found in tap water.

WELL WATER: Most spring and well waters are not much better than tap water. The minerals in most wells are cationic in nature.

Very few wells contain beneficial anionic minerals such as potassium or sodium sulfate. Statistically people who drink from these wells are much healthier than people who drink from wells that contain cationic charged minerals.

Well owners have another problem to deal with in that industrial waste chemicals are seeping into soils and polluting deep aquafers. In Arizona, which is noted for its pure well water, most wells have been shown to contain TCE, a powerful industrial solvent that is carcinogenic.

B0TTLED WATER: Bottled waters fall into several types:

1. Spring Water, 2. Manufactured Water, 3. Distilled Water, 4. Naturally Carbonated, 5. Artificially Carbonated.

Most bottled mineral waters are manufactured by first removing the natural minerals and contaminants by means of reverse osmosis and/or deionization. Mineral free water is then made into mineral water by addition of mineral salts which are meant to give water good taste.

Bottling companies that do this are not aware of the effects of cationic and anionic minerals on blood zeta potential. As a result most of these waters are not good for us.

The spring waters of Europe are natural mineral waters that contain various percentages of cationic and anionic minerals. Most bottled mineral waters contain an imbalance of electrolytes and are decidedly cationic.

The only one that appears to be anionic is Volvic Water from France.

DISTILLED WATER: Given a choice of the above waters, we would choose distilled water over cationic water. This is because it does not disturb the charge on colloids in the blood system.

Of course, the very best water is distilled water to which high zeta colloids have been added. These are contained in Crystal Energy Concentrate™

CARB0NATED BEVERAGES: Carbon Dioxide gas, or CO_2, is added to water to produce sparkling-water and club soda. In the human body, carbon dioxide is a deadly waste product of metabolism, it is carried by the blood to the lungs where it is exchanged for incoming oxygen and then expelled with the outgoing breath.

The average adult exhales enough carbon dioxide and other poisons of metabolism in a 24-hour period to kill 12 adult elephants. Carbon dioxide is a deadly gas. Great numbers of people have died from CO_2 poisoning. As this gas is heavier than air, it sinks to low places like sewers and well bottoms. There are many cases on record where people have gone down into an old well and died instantly from excess carbon dioxide gas. The recent thousands of people who died in Cameroon are a testament to the toxic effect of carbon dioxide.

The Earth's atmosphere contains 0.04% CO_2. If the content were increased to 3% all life would become unconscious. If increased to 4% all animal and insect life would die. For this reason it is extremely important to ventilate our homes and bedrooms. Every person needs 3,000 cubic feet of fresh air per hour.

When we drink highly carbonated beverages we increase the amount of CO_2 gas in our blood streams and place a heavy load on our gaseous waste handling system.

The increased load of CO_2 decreases our ability to handle oxygen.

When carbon dioxide combines with water it creates carbonic acid which plays a vital role in nature. This. acid decomposes limestone and other minerals and makes these available to plants.

Carbonated water will make your plants grow vigorously but is not good for us to drink.

Micro-organisms in the first few feet of soil release carbon dioxide as part of their metabolism. his creates a pressure in the soil that causes the creation of carbonic acid when rain water trickles through soil layers. The carbonic acid in turn dissolves minerals which are then picked up by plants and used for food.

The excess minerals wash into streams and are used by aquatic life.

ALCOHOLIC BEVERAGES

In a colloid system a moderate amount of alcohol will give a slight increase in zeta potential, beyond that an increased percentage of alcohol causes a massive coagulation of these particles.

The ratio of good to bad alcohol percentage is critical.

Our bodies manufacture a small amount of alcohol for biological purposes.

Beer is extremely harmful to the system because it contains large amounts of cationic electrolytes. The beer industry uses the hardest water it can find, and then adds large quantities of cationic minerals to its brewing water.

As a result, beer may be more harmful than other alcoholic beverages.

The wine industry sometimes filters its wine through asbestos filters. Tiny particles of asbestos may get into the wine, and as we know asbestos is a powerful carcinogen.

COFFEE AND TEA

We have not tested the effects of caffeine or coffee on zeta potential. However, caffeine is a powerful drug that causes the release of adrenalin into the blood stream. Most drug alkaloids are cationic and therefore are destructive to colloid stability.

After using Crystal Energy Concentrate™ for a year, we have completely eliminated caffeine from our diet. Our increase in natural energy and well-being was enormous.

CLOTHES

Natural fibers have a neutral or slightly positive charge. This causes the person who wears them to attract negative ions to their bodies.

Negative ions are then inhaled into the respiratory tract where they increase charge on blood colloids.

Plastic clothes like polyesters and acrylics on the other hand have a high voltage negative charge associated with them. This negative charge attracts positive ions or pollutants from the air into the environment of the body.

These pollutants are inhaled into the respiratory system where they are damaging as they tend to destroy colloid stability.

Have you ever noticed that some people seem to attract cigarette smoke? Smoke is positively charged. It is attracted to negatively charged clothes. People who, wear polyester leisure suits attract more pollutants to their bodies.

SALT AND OTHER SPICES

As discussed previously, salt (sodium chloride) is not a necessary ingredient for the diet. We get enough sodium in natural foods. Food processors and restaurants add tremendous amounts of salt to food in order to enhance flavor.

Monosodium glutamate is another culprit. Many restaurants, especially oriental restaurants, add it to their food to act as a flavor enhancer. It is actually a preservative and acts to keep their dishes bacteria-free for weeks on end without refrigeration. Many of these places keep aluminum pots full of MSG-treated foods. When the customer orders a dish they simply add these together, heat them and serve.

MSG is the cause of Chinese Restaurant Syndrome which is a type of migraine headache caused by MSG. In the Orient they call it AJINOMOTO because Japan's Ajinomoto Chemical Company is the world's largest manufacturer of monosodium glutamate.

CHAPTER 13

HOW IS CRYSTAL ENERGY CONCENTRATE" MADE?

Crystal Energy Concentrate™ or CEC is made in the laboratory. These high zeta potential colloids are synthesized by an almost alchemical process. All the ingredients used in the colloid synthesis are United States Pharmaceutical Grade. This means that the items used are extremely pure and have been approved for use in the manufacture of food products and drugs. We might add that all the ingredients used in the manufacture of Crystal Energy Concentrate™ are found in mother's milk. The quantities of the various ingredients in our product are well below that allowed for use in food products. ALL THE INGREDIENTS USED IN THE MANUFACTURE OF OUR COLLOIDS ARE FOUND NATURALLY IN FRESH FRUITS AND BERRIES.

The list of ingredients on the label reads: Distilled Water, Silica, Potash, Soda, Magnesium Chloride, and Excipients. When these ingredients are combined in a specific way, they create a multimineral colloidal polysilicate of high electric charge or zeta potential. As chemical names tend to upset some of us, let's take a look at the ingredients:

1. Distilled water: In the manufacture of these colloids it is necessary to use the highest purity water. In the delicate phase of colloid formation any impurities would interfere with the production of colloids—of the desired quality.

2. Silica: Silica is amorphous silicon dioxide. Silica is the most abundant element in the entire universe. It is found in abundance in the human body and is found in all vegetation. Silica is found in great concentration in the Heavenly Horsetail herb. Pure silica is used, as the basis of our colloids.

3. Potash: This is a crude name for a fraction of the purified ash of vegetable fibers. This is an alkaline potassium ash which has been purified. Potash is found as the alkali ne element in fruits such as oranges and bananas.

4. Soda: Soda Ash is also an alkaline sodium compound which may also obtained from a fraction of the ashes of vegetables and fruits.

5. Magnesium Chloride: Magnesium Chloride is found in great quantities in sea water and is also found in fruits and vegetables. Magnesium is one of the most important elements in the human body. Magnesium chloride is a catalyst.

6. Excipients: Excipients are trace ingredients that are also a trade secret. We can say that these elements are found naturally in fruits and berries. These ingredients are listed on the GRAS list (Generally Regarded As Safe) and include the organic polymer coating that protects our colloids from discharging their electric field. Albuminoids act in the same way in the protection of colloids in vegetable juices.

The above ingredients are combined in a slow and tedious process. This process involves 31 steps from beginning to completion and takes three days. Some of the steps involve heating and cooling to certain precise temperatures.

When the colloids are formed, they have a certain electric charge or zeta potential. After the product is formed it is then placed in a device of our invention which is known as a Tangential Vortex Amplifier, This device creates a perfect vortex structure which, when combined with an electronic field device, greatly raises the charge on the colloids. When the charge has reached its peak, the colloids are coated with a thin film of organic polymer to insulate against discharge.

The manufacturing technique is really an analog of the technique used by mother nature in the production of colloids in Hunza water. As glacier water runs down the sides of the mountains it picks up speed and comes crashing down into ancient mineral fields where it picks up its silicate colloidal minerals The ancient mineral field also contains an organic polymer that coats the colloids and acts as an insulator to help prevent discharge. The turbulent motion of the water also creates millions of vortexes that charge the colloids with energy. These vortexes are energized by magnetic fields and high altitude. ultra-violet light rays. Unfortunately, there are only five places on Earth where these things happen naturally, and all these places are virtually inaccessible.

The quantity of colloids required to alter the surface tension of water is extremely low. By the time these are diluted for drinking the total amount added to water is on the order of 4 parts per million. This means that 4 milligrams (0.004 grams) of colloids are added 'per liter of drinking water.

When this quantity of colloids is added to distilled water the resulting surface tension is between 55 and 65. Which is well below the surface tension of Hunza water which is 68. The process of manufacturing Crystal Energy Concentrate™ is so complex that it cannot be duplicated outside our laboratories.

TO SUMMARIZE

Crystal Energy Concentrate™ colloids are multi-mineral colloidal polysilicates.

These colloids are protected or insulated against loss of charge by means of an organic polymeric adsorbed coating that is much stable than albumin.

Depending on concentration, we can reduce the surface tension of water from its normal 73 dynes to 26 dynes per centimeter.

As these colloids increase the formation of liquid crystals in water, it may be that water so structured is similar to the water found in normal tissue fluids.

USES FOR CRYSTAL ENERGY CONCENTRATE™

The high energy colloidal silicates which we have developed behave in the same way as the Hunza colloids except our colloids have a much higher zeta potential.

When we drank large quantities of these colloids, the surface tension of our urine dropped from' 68 to 45 in just one hour! This was associated with an increase in physical energy.

We have been drinking these highly charged colloids now for two and one half years.

These colloids are now in use by Olympic Gold Medalists, Mr. Olympia body builders, race horses, farmers, and many health minded people all over the world.

Most people begin by drinking two glasses of Crystal Activated Water™ per day for the first week thereafter increasing the amount by one glass per day per week 2 until all water consumed is activated.

OTHER USES INCLUDE:

1. CUT FLOWERS: Add 20 drops of the concentrate to a vase of cut flowers. The flowers will remain fresh much longer. Spray foliage with 1 oz/gal mix every day.

2. VEGETABLE AND FRUIT WASH: Add one ounce of the concentrate to 32 oz. of distilled water and use as a fruit and vegetable wash (1 oz. per quart). It is best to apply this solution by means of a spray bottle.

3. SPROUTS AND GARDENING: For delicious juicy sprouts, soak seeds in a one ounce per gallon dilution and water daily with the same solution. For farming, spray the seeds with activated water before planting. For transplanting, spray roots and soil with water before replacing dirt.

4. SUNBATHING: Put the 1 oz/gal. mix into a spray bottle and spray it on exposed parts of the body. Spray once every half hour or whenever the need arises.

5. COOKING: use the 1 oz/gal mix when making coffee, tea, or herbal beverages. The reduced surface tension will increase the extraction efficiency. Also use it wherever water is called for, for example in making spaghetti or rice.

6. HOUSEPLANTS: Water once with Crystal water and then water with CEC once a week and use regular water in between. Also, mist the leaves with Crystal Activated Water (1 oz/gal) once a week.

7. SHAMPOO: Add one ounce of CEC (Crystal Energy Coneentrate™) to nine ounces of shampoo for more luxuriant lather. CEC can also be added to dish washer detergent as well as to laundry detergent.

8. BATHING: Add one cup of 1 oz/gal mix to a bathtub full of water. Add one cup of same to your spa or hot tub. Add one ounce of CEC to nine ounce of liquid bath soap.

9. TEETH: Brush your teeth with a 1 oz/gal mix.

10. SHAVING: For a super clean and smooth shave, spray the 1 oz/ gal mix on your beard.

11. RACE HORSES: Treat 1/2 of the daily water consumption with CEC. This usually amounts to 5 gallons of water per day.

12. PETS: Shampoo your pets with CEC diluted into shampoo as above' It gives their coats a healthy sheen and helps to keep fleas and. ticks away. Add CEC to your pet's drinking water, they love it.

CHAPTER 14

HOW WE ENHANCE OUR
ZETA POTENTIAL

FIRST: We drink at least 8 glasses of Crystal Energy Concentrate™ every day. The high energy colloids are the foundation upon which we build our life.

SECOND: We have eliminated all dietary factors which, destroy colloidal stability. These include the elimination of stimulants such as coffee, tea, alcohol and animal products from our diet. This also includes the elimination of cooked food. Since a large number of cations are found in polluted air, we make it a point to always spend our time in healthy fresh moving air. Our home is well ventilated in summer and winter and has numerous electric fans to ensure air circulation. Still air, like still water, grows stagnant and poisonous. We live in a country environment that is free of pollution and do not allow ourselves to be in the same environment as a smoker.

To ensure that the air in our home is free of airborne contaminants we use another invention of ours, the EFG or Electron Field Generator. This device utilizes a newly discovered electronic field effect to eliminate toxins from the environment. It is the best air purifier available today anywhere in the world.

THIRD: We exercise every day to enhance the flow of nutrients to our cells, and to facilitate the removal of toxins from our bodies.

FOURTH: We spice our foods with our Herbal Enlightenment blend which is composed of special longevity herbs and spices. These are dried at low temperatures to retain the stability of the albuminoids which coat these natural colloids.

FIFTH: We eat a very pure diet free of refined (dead) foods. Our current diet is composed of fresh raw fruits with a few vegetables. We eat no animal products at all.

SIXTH: We drink a lot of fresh raw vegetables juices. These juices are full of high zeta colloids and anionic electrolytes.

Carrot juice is especially full of these elements. As mentioned in earlier chapters, the surface tension of fresh carrot juice is 30.

SEVENTH: We take air and sun baths every day. We take our baths before 11 in the morning and after 2 in the afternoon. We also spend a lot time in our hot tub spa to which we have added a substantial amount of Crystal Energy Concentrate™.

Although we believe a simple lifestyle is very important, the use of Crystal Energy Concentrate™ cannot be overemphasized. CEC is the result of. 24 years of research on our part, which was the result of nearly 60 years of research which was begun by Dr. Henri Coanda the father. of fluid dynamics.

Even if our dietary recommendations are too rigorous for 99% of our readers we would urge you to include in your daily diet as much raw fruit as possible. Raw sprouts such as mung bean and alfalfa are also loaded with high zeta colloids.

As high zeta potential colloids are consumed your energy level will go up and your body will become alive with new vibrant energy. This influx of life will begin to re-sensitize your system to what is good for it. The path is automatic. All you have to do is take that first step.

APPENDIX A

Reader's Digest, March 1936

Condensed from Rockefeller Center Weekly 01935, Center Publications, Inc., 30 Rockefeller Plaza, N.Y.C. (Rockefeller Center Weekly, October 31, 1935)

Reader's Digest, March 1936

A group of executives sat tense and silent in an office in the RCA Building in New York City. They stared with incredulous eyes at a purple orchid. A short time before it had been rescued from a pile of debris, a withered, yellowed thing, dead. Now the petals were fresh and crisp, its color vivid. It was blooming with new life, and would continue to do so for 16 or 17 days!

Dr. Frederick S. Macy, one of the country's outstanding bacteriologists, had added a teaspoonful of an amber-tinted liquid to a quart of water in the bottle which held the flower. Here was striking indication of the mysteries that lie ahead in the comparatively unexplored realm of science known as colloidal chemistry. It was one of innumerable experiments these gentlemen had been witnessing for a year or more, on behalf of their internationally known pharmaceutical company. A few days later they signed an 18-year contract for the rights to a solution similar to the one in Dr. Macy's bottle. They will invest more than $2,000,000 a year in it from now on.

To gain a working conception of what colloidal chemistry is, consider that fiving tissues and organs are simply great masses of cells—billions of them. The energy, the very life-force of these cells is obtained from certain minerals and metals, among them iron, iodine, manganese, copper. There are some 32, with traces of as many others, in the human body. colloidal chemistry is the science which converts those elements into particles so minute that they can be utilized by living cells.

Normally nature supplies the cells with these elements in their colloidal form. Science has now learned to produce these colloids in the laboratory. Lately, life has been prolonged by colloid action," says Dr. Macy, "and better knowledge of the subject will certainly result in prolonging the normal term of existence." In the case of the apparently dead orchid, copper in colloidal form was needed to restore the proper balance of the mineral and metals that comprised the life cells of the flower. Once that balance was restored, the cells began to function and the orchid lived again.

In the Colloidal Laboratories of America they have a motion picture which is as weird as anything ever shown on a screen a movie of a headache. The actors are the nerves in a human head magnified millions of times. you see the headache. Those nerve endings are tangled, twisting, writhing. Then you see the colloids enter. These rescuers, smaller than the blood corpuscles themselves, march straight to the spot where there is an unbalance of the vital metals. You see those laboratory prepared colloids restore normalcy there at the seat of the trouble. Then you see the nerves cease their twisting, relax and assume their proper position.

Dr. Steinmetz, the wizard of electricity, devised a method of utilizing colloids in the treatment of sinus trouble. The Bide a Wee Home, New York's famous hospital for cats and dogs, can cure mange in three days, where it used to take three months. A large midwestern city was freed from the scourge of goiter when colloidal iodine was added to the water supply. A famous institution for the treatment of alcoholism is experimenting with a colloidal solution which apparently not only overcomes the effects of excessive drinking but removes the craving for liquor as well. Such treatment consists of the introduction of metals—gold and iodine, in the case of alcoholism--which correct the unbalance caused by alcoholic poisons.

The effect of colloids is explainable in part by electric action. Sick and dead and broken down cells are attracted to the colloids by electro-magnetic force, as iron filings are attracted to a magnet. The colloids carry those decayed or poisonous substances into the bloodstream, and they are eliminated, the system meanwhile adapting what it needs of the colloids.

A simple illustration will suggest the immense powers that are being unsealed. Suppose we have a cube of iron measuring an inch on each edge. The total surface would be six square inches. The electrical charge is on the surface;

therefore, the greater the surface the greater the charge; and if we divide the cube of iron into smaller pieces we increase the surface areas. By colloidal chemistry, that iron cube can be divided into particles so minute that that they are invisible, hence instead of six square inches of surface emanating electric energy, we have something like 127 acres.

In colloidal form iodine, for example, is one of the elements essential for the well-being of human cells. yet if you should drink as much as two or three grains of free iodine, it would kill you. Dr. Macy, when explaining this, held up an eight-ounce cup full of colloidal iodine. "There," he said, "is the equivalent of 740 grains of free iodine— enough to kill 300 men." And he drank it. In that form, iodine is not only harmless, but beneficial. The same is true of arsenic and other deadly poisons.

Colloidal chemistry was evolved by David Graham, a British chemist, 50 years ago, but only recently has it been-realized, even by scientists, what an enormous influence it is destined to have in medicine, agriculture, industry. "We have television now," one of the world's greatest scholars said recently. "There is, as I see it just one great development left for our time. That is the 'Fourth Estate of Matter,' the other three being land, water and air."

Says Dr. Macy: "The study of these phenomena constitutes the road to the ultimate in human knowledge."

APPENDIX B

CRYSTAL ENERGY CONCENTRATE™
WHAT IS IT?

Crystal Energy Concentrate is a colloidal trace mineral silicate of high zeta potential or electrical charge. This mineral is a physical analog of the trace mineral silicates found in areas where people live to be in excess of 100 years. Areas like Hunzaland in the Karakorum mountains of Tibet, the Vilacabamba of Ecuador, and the county of Georgia in the Soviet Union. Crystal Energy Concentrate™ is the culmination of 24 years of research by Dr. Patrick Flanagan, proclaimed as one of America's top ten scientists by LIFE magazine and his co-researcher/wife, Gael Crystal Flanagan.

Colloids are known as the 'twilight zone of matter.' These minerals are the smallest particles that matter can be divided while still maintaining its individual characteristics. colloids range in size from 0.01 millionths of an inch to 10 millionths of an inch (.01 microns to 10 microns). The smaller colloids cannot be seen with the most powerful microscopes. Because of their small size, they have an enormous surface area which gives them special properties. One teaspoon of colloids can have a total surface area of over 127 acres, and is composed of billions of tiny electrically charged minerals.

Colloids of high electrical charge are found outside the living system naturally only in special places like those mentioned above.

Crystal Energy Concentrate™ is made in our laboratory by a secret process that first creates these particles from United States Pharmaceutical Grade minerals. Once these colloids are created, they are given a powerful electrical charge by means of a device which is known as a Tangential Vortex Amplifier. This device imparts an electro-magnetic inductive high potential charge on each colloidal particle; This high energy charge is measured in millivolts and is known as zeta potential. The potential on each of our colloids averages 125 millivolts = 0.125 volts. This potential which is known as zeta potential may not seem like much, however if we have 1,000,000 colloids in a glass of water, the total electric charge in that glass is 1,000,000 X 0.125 volts or 125,000 volts!

To gain a working conception of what colloidal chemistry is, consider that living tissues, and organs are simply great masses of cells—billions of them. The energy, the very life-force of these cells, is obtained from certain minerals and metals, among them iron, iodine, manganese, copper. There are some 32, with traces of as many others in the human body. Colloidal chemistry is the science which converts those elements into particles so minute that they can be utilized by living cells.

The effect of colloids is explainable in part by electric action. Sick and dead and broken down cells are attracted to the colloids by electro-magnetic force, as iron filings are

94

attracted to a magnet. The colloids carry those decayed or poisonous substances into the bloodstream, and they are eliminated, the system meanwhile adapting what it needs of the colloids.

COLLOIDS AND WATER

Water is the basis of all life. The human body is composed on the average of approximately 75% water. The brain can be as high as 75%. water. Even bones have 68% water. The water in the living system is not the same as water found in lakes, ponds and oceans. The water in the living system is a highly structured living liquid crystal.

Bulk water, or water outside the living system is a sea of molecular chaos and normally has very little structure. A glass sf ordinary water is composed mostly of random oriented water molecules. There is however a tiny percentage of liquid crystals (structured water) in ordinary water. These liquid crystals are like tiny icebergs floating in a sea of chaos.

In the living system, a great percentage of water is of the liquid crystal type. When we drink water, the body must take the sea of chaos and convert it into a liquid crystal before it can be used in the living cell. This structuring is done by means of colloidal minerals and enzymes which are ingested by eating raw food or in the case of Hunzaland also come from the special high energy colloidal water which is found in the river there. When raw food is cooked or processed, the colloids are denatured. That is, they lose their electrical charge and coagulate—they are dead.

When our Crystal Energy Concentrate™ trace minerals are added to ordinary water, the millions of tiny electrically charged colloidal particles each act as a seed for the growth of a liquid crystal. These tiny negatively charged particles form a nucleus of energy which attracts water molecules and is therefore an electrical center for the formation of structured water.

As the percentage of liquid crystals increase, the physical properties of water change. One of the most important indicators of liquid crystal water is shown by a reduction in surface tension. It is the reduction of surface tension of structured water that enables it to act as a powerful detoxifier and transporter of cellular nutrients. Since Crystal Energy Concentrate™ is already structured, the living system does not need to use valuable, energy reserves to restructure the bulk water when it is consumed.

A number of environmental antagonists tend to de-structure the water in living systems. The consumption of processed and cooked foods, stress, electromagnetic pollution (ELF waves), toxins, drugs, and unnatural chemical compounds all tend to destroy the change on bio-colloids. When the charge is reduced energy is low and the body cannot eliminate its accumulating toxins. These toxins and then stored in various places for eventual elimination if and when the condition is relieved.

USES FOR CRYSTAL ENERGY CONCENTRATE™

While no medical claims are made or implied for Crystal Energy Concentrate™ users unanimously report a significant increase in energy and feelings of well-being.

This high energy colloidal concentrate has been used by world class Olympic athletes, race horses, champion body builders, and ordinary people who wish to improve their state of well-being.

No claims are made for this product for the diagnosis, treatment, or mitigation of any disease or disease condition. The purchaser agrees that no medical claims are made or shall be made for this product.

APPENDIX C

REPORT ON CRYSTAL ENERGY CONCENTRATE-
By Dr. Michael Hopping

There are a large and growing number of people who are enthusiastically claiming to have found an "edge" or advantage over those who have not found it yet.

Over one year ago I started 'to investigate this phenomenon. My reaction is that in my quarter century of intense interest in maximizing human performance, never before have I seen such a pronounced beneficial effect on so many people in such diverse applications as when they are influenced by Crystal Energy Concentrate™.

Since no attempt is made to claim medical or therapeutic cures with it, all credit must apparently be given to the normalizing or potentiating of performances.

The most obvious persons to appreciate this boost are athletes, simply because they are already at the edge of their peak performance and can easily assess the advantage they experience over previous lifetime best efforts. There must be sound reasons for the fact that there are an emerging number of serious athletes, professional and amateur, benefiting from it.

To eliminate the possibility of any placebo or psychological factor in evaluating it, several thoroughbred race horses have benefited from its use during middle to long-term testing. Careful monitoring of blood and urine demonstrates no problems to these equine athletes while speed and stamina are raised by 4 - 5 body lengths per 6 furlongs by the end of the first month, and up to 10 - 11 body lengths by the end oi the second month. This equates to an additional 90+ feet of distance covered in the same amount of time. Human athletes, coaches and trainers have no difficulty in understanding this value to them.

The rest of us enjoy the relief from being tired so much of the time. Another asset is that, since it is not a drug or CNS stimulant such as caffeine, there is no uncomfortable zizz and therefore no subsequent lag. Rather than extreme highs and lows, an enhanced norm is experienced. It is easier to accomplish more work than usual.

To explain some of how this happens, first realize that the human body is about 70% water, and the brain is over 80% water content. Now picture a pan of water being heated. As it reaches boiling there is great movement until the point where the water molecules leap up into the air with the increase in energy. Now suppose that instead of heat energy being applied to the pan of water, electrical energy were used.

The naked eye could not see the change, nor would there be a temperature increase. The water molecules would respond to the additional energy by transforming the hydrogen bond pattern from H_2O monomers into $(H_2O)_6$ octomers, possessing vastly different properties. When swallowed, these effects are then utilizable in supporting life and vitality instead of being wasted as in the case with heat energy.

One of the most celebrated and encouraging scientific works of our century has been the work of Dr. Alexis Carrel. Dr. Carrel, working at the Rockefeller Institute, won the Nobel Prize in medicine by demonstrating this arresting hypothesis: "The cell is immortal. It is merely the fluid in which it floats which degenerates. Renew the fluid at intervals, give the cells what they require for nutrition and, as far as we know, the pulsation of life may go on forever. He won that coveted award by keeping a chicken heart vibrantly alive and functioning for a full 20 years before ending the experiment.

In a completely independent pursuit, but perfectly complimenting this work, Dr. Patrick Flanagan sought additional answers to the mysteries of extending life and vitality.

Flanagan was a child prodigy who had earned acclaim in several venues of physics through a series of patented inventions used by various agencies of our Federal government.

His worldwide patents on such diverse contributions as the most effective air purifier in use today anywhere, the hearing aid for the totally deaf, various speech synthesizers, monitoring devices for examining force fields and others placed him in the category of a maximum contributor to the quality of life in our time. Dr. Flanagan traveled the world, conferring with those who were already experiencing enviably healthy lives in significant concentrations. He examined their lives and tested their nutrients and waters using parameters of both chemistry and physics. He monitored a definite, measurable electrical change within the waters from Hunzaland, for example.

A similar observation was noted with the waters from Lourdes in France, Baden-Baden in Germany and other sites known for centuries as possessing unusually beneficial properties. He then returned to America where he applied rigorous methodologies aimed at deliberately replicating and then improving both the effect and the stability of the charge carrying colloidal dispersants within those waters from afar. Flanagan tested the full range of vegetables, fruits and grains to determine the optimal properties of the life-giving enzymes found in nature.

Enzymes are colloidal dispersants. Blood is a colloidal dispersant. Human mothers' milk is a colloidal dispersant. And so forth. In addition to the unusual measurements, he also measured the surface tension and zeta potential (net electrical charge on the solid particles within a colloid of each. He noted that optimal[1] health was enhanced in direct proportion to the amount of zeta potential and in inverse proportion to the level of surface tension.

Hence, the first monumental breakthrough that the higher zeta potential and lower surface tension within limits, the better.

For example, freshly juiced carrot juice was found to have the highest zeta potential, approximately 38 millivolts, and the lowest surface tension, sometimes as low as 30 dynes/cm. It is presumably very supportive of life at that time. But these attributes were of short duration because both were lost in only 24 hours.

The next day carrot juice looked and tasted the same, but had lost the coveted physics advantages entirely. So stability of the colloidal dispersion was found to be of immense importance.

These advantages seem to extend and mirror the desirable effects of the 5,000 or so enzymes giving life to each human body.

It then took many years to resolve the secrets of optimizing the stability of the highly charged colloidal dispersion. Only then did Dr. Flanagan widen his circle of co-laboring peers within the scientific community.

These scientists continue to use the inelastic neutron scanners, x-ray diffraction scanners, infrared spectrometers, zetameters, ring surface tensiometers, dark field microscope systems such as Live Cell analysis, Voll meters, Viscometers, ultraviolet spectrometers, Nuclear Magnetic Resonance spectrometers to document discernible differences.

The rest of us in the world do not need any such testing to notice how much better we feel. And only now for the first time can we make this known to those around us.

This gives us a stable platform for this gratifying offering. The benefits extend through our families to those around us. We then share the significance of Dr. Flanagan's work, extending his huge contribution to mankind.

Since we reap what we sow in this Life we may expect a thrilling harvest to our lives.

APPENDIX D

HEALTH AND MEDICAL OBSERVAT.IONS FOR CRYSTAL ENERGY CONCENTRATE™

PREPARATION OF COLLOIDAL MINERALS

By Martin Dayton, M.D.

ABBREVIATED CURRICULUM VITAE

Dr. Martin Dayton

Dr. Dayton practices family, general and holistic medicine in North Miami Beach, Florida, U.S.A. He has a B.S. degree in research a D.O. degree with board certification in general medicine; and a D.D. degree with board certification in family practice. He is completing his Ph.D. degree in electrical acupuncture and is a licensed homeopathic physician. In addition to being a member of the American Medical Association and American Osteopathic Association, he has credentials involving various Holistic, Homeopathic, Nutritional, Preventive, and acupuncture organizations. Dr. Dayton teaches medical and osteopathic students and doctors and has clinical faculty disappointments. His patients include local, national and international clientele. Dr. Dayton lectures in the United States and abroad.

INTRODUCTION

I am honored to have the opportunity to work with Crystal Energy Concentrate™ before it had a name. Crystal Energy Concentrate™ had been first introduced to me as a colloidal formulation of mineral silicates created through the genius of Patrick Flanagan, Ph.D., and his wife co-researcher, Gael Crystal Flanagan. Prior to being made aware of Dr. Flanagan's formulation, I had researched health claims made for colloidal mineral waters. I was familiar with several colloidal mineral preparations produced commercially. I was familiar with Dr. Flanagan's reputation and was fascinated with energy related devices he has produced in the past. When I was approached to investigate the potential usefulness of a not yet marketed colloidal formulation created by Dr. Flanagan, I was intrigued. I was put in contact with Dr. Flanagan. Our conversation on the physical and chemical properties of Crystal Energy Concentrate™, left me enlightened and enthusiastic. Unable to resist temptation, I embarked on what is still an ongoing investigative adventure.

I wish to share with you in the following text a few of our observations of this adventure. These observations have led to theories of the effect of Crystal Energy Concentrate on human health and well-being.

TEXT

One of my first observations of Crystal Energy Concentrate™ involved spraying it on freshly sunburned skin contact with the spray consistently brought almost instantaneous relief of pain. without adverse side effects. The phenomenon appeared so predictable that I bragged to friends who were getting a bit well done at an ocean swimming party. Expecting to be hailed as a hero, I sprayed the sunburned areas on my friends and myself. To my embarrassment everyone experienced more pain. Suspecting a mix up in the liquid used we washed with fresh water. The burning subsided to a pre-spraying intensity. Not finding any mix ups, I timidly re-sprayed. The pain was relieved as it had been shown to do so in the past.

In search of an explanation, I reviewed the sequence of events. The first time I had sprayed salt from drying ocean water had accumulated on our sunburned skin. Burns are a form of wounds. Perhaps the concentrate had caused the salt to penetrate the wounded skin more easily. The increased pain may have been due to a pouring salt into an open wound effect Perhaps the concentrate increases the ease with which substances can penetrate and travel through the involved tissues.

Pain may occur when an impaired ability exists to transport materials necessary for normal function and repair to areas where they are needed. Pain may occur also when an impaired ability exists to transport toxic materials, which prevent normal function and repair, from areas where they accumulate. In sunburn both these impairments exist. Rapid formulation of toxic substances, swelling and compromised circulation impair transportation of the materials.

Improving transportation may speed healing and reduce pain. The concentrate may reduce pain through improved transportation of materials through the body's tissues. Enhancement of transportation explains both the observations of worsening pain when salt is present and improvement of pain when salt is not present.

Another dramatic observation was made while I attended a demonstration of 'dark field' microscopy in analysis of whole blood. 'Dark field' microscopy shows the activity of live cells and other structures in freshly drawn blood. Among the constituents in the blood are small disk-like structures called erythrocytes or red blood cells. These cells are designed to transport oxygen and nutrients throughout the body. As red blood cells are slightly larger than our capillaries, they must be discrete, that is, they must flow freely and individually in order to reach all the cells of the body. Red blood cells have a diameter of 8.5 microns while capillaries have an average inside diameter of 6 microns. If these cells are clumped or stuck together they cannot flow and circulation is impaired. When red blood cells do not aggregate into clumps, blood flows more easily.

During the demonstration, a young lady doctor who was having her menstrual period stated she was having a pounding headache. She explained that pounding headaches were regularly associated with her menstruation. The doctor conducting the demonstration noted that clumping is more prevalent during times of menstruation. The doctor further noted that clumping may impair circulation in smaller blood vessels leading to headaches.

We took a sample of the menstruating doctor's blood and observed it under the 'dark field' microscope. Indeed, there was prominent clumping. In the interest of science, the menstruating doctor drank a half ounce of undiluted Crystal Energy Concentrate™ The headache disappeared within two minutes. Her blood was immediately tested under the microscope. The prominent clumping was no longer seen.

To determine if this observation was a coincidence, I selected several male doctors at the medical convention. All demonstrated excessive clumping in their blood. Obviously excessive blood clumping is not exclusively due to menstruation. Each was given the concentrate. The blood clumping normalized within minutes on retesting for all the doctors evaluated. The Crystal Energy Concentrate™ can decrease excessive blood clumping.

Through Dr. Flanagan, I was made aware of a race horse which bled whenever it ran. These horses are called bleeders due to weak capillaries in their lungs. After being given the concentrate on a daily basis, the horse no longer bled when it raced. I gave the concentrate to another race horse that also had bleeding tendencies when racing. After two weeks on the concentrate the horse came in on the money without bleeding problems.

If the concentrate helps avoid excessive clumping on one hand, and also stops excessive bleeding on the other, is it possible that it acts to balance and stabilize the circulatory system? The living system is programmed for self- preservation. part of this programming is to select nutrients that help to protect the system from imbalance.

To observe the immediate effects of the concentrate, electromagnetic instruments may be helpful. To observe the effects on general balance of the body an electromagnetic measurement device, the Japanese Ryodoraku neurometer may be employed. The Ryodoraku neurometer measures the electromagnetic activity of 24 acupuncture points on the body.

The measurements are plotted on a graph to determine disturbances in energy field balance. Using the graph of measurements, often patients' symptoms can be deter-mined with an amazing degree of accuracy, without the benefit of a prior history.

The research on the Ryodoraku neurometer measurements are based on many thousands of eases. The measurements are thought to reflect the state of the autonomic nervous system and acupuncture meridian balance. As suspected, the measurement results via the Ryodoraku neurometer reflected the improvement of energy balance when the concentrate was used.

To observe the near instantaneous effects of Crystal Energy Concentrate™ on individual parts of the body electromagnetically, a German E.A.V.-inspired device may be employed. This device measures changes in energy fields of specific organs and body areas through electrical acupuncture point measurement. Similar to the Ryodoraku neurometer, the E.A.V.-inspired device is backed by extensive experience and research. Again, as suspected, the measurement results of the E.A.V.-inspired device reflected improvement in energy balance when the concentrate was used.

Such devices have been found useful in the clinical practice of electroacupuncture and homeopathy worldwide. Both electroacupuncturists and homeopaths approach disease by correcting imbalances in a person's energy fields. The electroacupuncturist stimulates points on the body with electricity and/or needles. The homeopath usually uses non-toxic energetically programmed medicines in liquid or solid form.

The energy devices are used to determine integrity of the energy fields of the body. The integrity of the energy field is thought to reflect the condition of the structures contained within the field. An abnormal energy field measurement may reflect a disease or tendency to disease before it becomes detectable by other means. Based on these findings, electro-acupuncturists and homeopaths therapeutically correct energy field disturbances, which are in turn reflected by beneficial physical and mental changes in an individual.

Observations of changes in energy balance seems to support the effectiveness of Crystal Energy Concentrate™. For example, I had a gratifying experience observing the improvement of an elderly lady who was a constipated arthritic with brittle nails surrounded by inflamed skin.

After taking the concentrate for several weeks her nails grew stronger and the inflammation subsided. This inflammation had been refractory to several topical medicines. Her arthritic discomfort lessened allowing for performance. Her constipation was relieved. She had a greater sense of well-being. After discontinuance of concentrate due to lack of supply, she worsened. After reinstitution, she improved again. At no time was her arthritis completely relieved and her joint deformities did not change. The effects were also not immediate.

Diseases are thought to reflect disharmony or imbalance in a person. If a person were perfectly balanced, by definition there would be no disease. If Crystal Energy Concentrate™ were to improve balance we might expect to see an improvement in physical signs and objective symptoms, when possible. this is indeed what happened. Crystal Energy Concentrate™ seems to promote health by improving body harmony and balance.

With great expectations, I made observations with other people. In spite of prejudicial optimism, not everybody felt better. Some showed little or no improvement. A few felt worse. Even people with seemingly similar conditions had different degrees of success.

How can this perplexing lack of predictability be explained? Perhaps Crystal Energy Concentrate™ affects people and their conditions in different ways depending on the underlying factors which contribute to their conditions.

Why would a few people seem not to improve? Perhaps symptoms or disease manifests when the sum total of underlying stressful factors outweigh the sum total of strengthening factors that resist the development of disease. In some instances the effects of Crystal Energy Concentrate™ may be insufficient.to help overcome a condition, resulting in no appreciable improvement.

The rapid release of toxic material stored in the body as a result of the effects large quantities of Crystal Energy Concentrate™ may conceivably trigger mild adverse symptoms. Such symptoms may come in the form of headaches, diarrhea, back ache, etc. These symptoms are known as cleansing reactions. Although transitory, they may be alleviated by decreasing the amount of concentrate taken per day.

Although Dr. Flanagan makes no claims for his product, some conditions were generally observed to fare better with the concentrate than others. For example, acne fared much better than psoriasis, which for the most part did not respond as satisfactorily as I would have liked. Arthritis had mixed results. Whether recommendations for administration were followed appropriately by any or all of the people whose conditions were observed is not known. Rigidly controlled studies were not performed. Apparently Crystal Energy Concentrate™ exerts a general action on the body. Variations in response are expected, being that each individual is unique and not quite like anyone else.

Other available methods for observation are numerous. All methods have relative advantages and disadvantages. Space permits the discussion of only a few methods to illustrate the efficacy of the theories discussed.

Theories are used to predict outcomes. They give us direction. They are often in need of modification as our knowledge expands. They guide us into the future.

Christopher Columbus before embarking on his famed journey, circa 1492, weighed the risks of sailing off the end of the world against the conclusions he drew from his own observations. The rest is history. Before embarking on a journey into future discoveries, we must determine risk. The amount of minerals present in Crystal Energy Concentrate™ measure well below United States government standard levels for toxicity. All the colloidal minerals found in the concentrate are of United States Pharmaceutical grade and are found on the GRAS list (Generally Regarded As Safe). In fact, the mineral level is far below that found in mineral waters such as Evian and Perrier. Thousands of people have taken the concentrate without any non-reversible or serious effects that I am aware.

THEORETICAL BENEFITS OF
CRYSTAL ENERGY CONCENTRATE™

The potential benefits and uses are numerous. We will address a few in the following paragraphs:

Crystal Energy Concentrate™ has a significant potential role in the field of nutrition by improving the absorption and assimilation of various nutritional substances. Reports of decreased bloating in some people when taking the concentrate are suggestive of improved absorption of substances from the gastrointestinal tract. A tendency for some people who have elevated levels of serum triglycerides (a type of fat found in the blood) to improve toward normalization when taking the concentrate is suggestive of improved assimilation of substances into the cells. Those with pre-existing impaired nutrition may most dramatically benefit from improved absorption and assimilation. Impaired nutritional states are more likely to occur with poorly balance diets, emotional stress, various disease states, and ageing. More sophisticated studies are needed.

Crystal Energy Concentrate™ may benefit various disease states which may result from biochemical deficiency and toxicity. Deficiency relates to not enough of appropriate material in any given area for optimal function and repair. Toxicity relates to too much inappropriate material in any given area which prevents optimal function and repair. By improving transportation, substances can reach areas where they are deficient and be removed from areas where they are in toxic excess.

Crystal Energy Concentrate™ may be used to address conditions which do not fall into disease categories. Conditions such as tiredness, restlessness or irritability may improve where no diagnosis is apparent. Some individuals have reported decreased tiredness, restlessness, and irritability while taking the concentrate.

The effects of Crystal Energy Concentrate™ may be helpful in attaining more optimal endurance and performance. The need for improved physical endurance and performance is not restricted to athletes. The effects of the concentrate may also be beneficial to improving mental performance and endurance as well.

ENERGY FIELD STABILIZATION

The energy field stabilization effect Crystal Energy Concentrate™ may have potential usefulness in health for everyone. While the study of bio-energy fields is a young science, the effect of the concentrate on the energy fields of the body may be profound. The work of Dr. Becker *et al* at 'the Upstate New York Veteran's hospital indicate that electric fields which are generated by injured tissues act to accelerate migration of ions and other nutrients to the damaged area. The electric charges on biological colloids may help to accelerate this process.

Those involved in the healing arts generally agree that the position of the physician is to provide the means whereby the body's forces may be balanced so that the body may activate its own healing functions.

Historically those civilizations which drank water with high colloidal mineral content are reputed to enjoy greater longevity and freedom from illness.

We would all hope that such would be the case for our own civilization. In laboratory studies, animal cells have been kept alive many times their normal expected lifespans by continuously replenishing of needed nutrients and cleansing of toxic materials.

NEEDED RESEARCH

Research is needed to determine the total effectiveness of Crystal Energy Concentrate™. The potential for human benefit may be great.

Research of this type is both expensive and time consuming. It may be a number of years before we realize the full potential of this great discovery.

DISCLAIMER

Not wishing to be accused of giving medical advice without proper patient examination and without appropriate local licensure, I cannot legally recommend taking Crystal Energy Coneentrate™ to anyone. For similar reasons I can not advocate not taking Crystal Energy Concentrate™ to anyone. I simply point out that theoretical potentials exist based on observations. Theoretical potentials should not be confused with claims and do not guarantee results.

Martin Dayton

Editor's Note: Crystal Energy Concentrate™ is a food beverage colloidal mineral water concentrate. When it is diluted for drinking it contains less than 3.9 parts per million of colloidal minerals. The popular French spring water, Evian, contains 481 parts per million in dissolved (non-colloidal) minerals. A 'Sante' water from Napa Valley, California contains 790 parts per million in dissolved minerals. One ounce of Crystal Energy Concentrate™ before dilution for drinking contains 469 parts per million of colloidal minerals. As the minerals in the concentrate are all U.S.P. grade, we can see that the concentration is far below that of some of the most popular spring waters that do not carry an electrical charge. The significance of the electrical charge on colloidal minerals is made obvious by this comparison. Even in minute quantities, the colloidal minerals in Crystal Energy Concentrate™ exert powerful effects.

APPENDIX E

THE AUTHORS

DR. PATRICK FLANAGAN is a scientist, inventor, researcher, award winning gymnast, humanitarian, pilot, and author of seven books, including the international best seller *Pyramid Power*. At the age: of 17, Dr. Flanagan was declared one of America's top ten scientists by LIFE Magazine.

Dr. Flanagan began his career as an electronics child prodigy. An amateur radio operator by the age of 8, he sold his first invention, a Guided Missile Detector to the U.S. Government when he was ll. At the age of 14 he invented the Neurophone, a hearing device that allows the deaf to hear, and enables direct programming of the long-term memory banks of the brain. By the age of 11 he was part of the Gemini Space Shot team and worked on the Gemini computer systems for NASA. At 23 he worked for the U.S. Navy and designed computers for translating human speech into Dolphin language for use in the Man-Dolphin communications program. He then moved into private research and has developed over 300 inventions, including the Electron Field Generator air purification system, and Crystal Energy Concentrate™, a colloidal energized mineral water.

He received his Doctor of Psychology degree from M.S.I.U. in 1972. In 1977 was made the Professor of Psychology and presented with the letters of Academicum Ex Classe Tibi Legitima of the prestigious Academia Gentium Pro-Pace in Rome, Italy. He has been listed in Leaders in American Science since 1962, and is the recipient of the Gold Plate Award presented by the American Academy of Achievement.

He has traveled around the world a number of times in search of secrets of revitalization and integration of the body's bio-energy systems.

GAEL CRYSTAL FLANAGAN: Gael, Dr. Patrick Flanagan's wife and co-researcher is a nationally known lecturer, writer, and nutritional consultant. She has spent a great part of the last two decades researching health modalities from around the world. She has been a total vegetarian for the past 18 years, and has developed a diet for maintaining perfect health.

She co-directed one of the country's first holistic health centers and has been a guest on numerous radio shows and has lectured on health throughout the country.

She is currently writing three books with Dr. Patrick Flanagan. Gael is also a physical fitness instructor, and teaches an exercise system which reverses the physical ageing process of the body. She specializes in the use of crystals for body healing and environmental enhancement.

Gael and Patrick recently received Doctor of Medicine degrees from the prestigious Medicina Alternativa in

Columbo, Sri Lanka. These degrees were issued at the Multi Disciplinary World Medical Congress.

Patrick and Gael were given the honor of being the first married couple in history to be in the King's Chamber of the Great Pyramid of Giza, Cairo, Egypt.

They presently live and work together in seclusion at their home in the mountains of Arizona.

NOTICE

The authors are in seclusion devoting their time to research and writing and as a result are not available for engagements, receive no visitors and grant no interviews. They cannot possibly answer all letters, but if any of the readers feel they must write, they may write to the authors care of the publisher which is the only way the authors can be contacted. The publisher has no authority to give anyone the address of the authors.

APPENDIX F

WATER FACTS

1. Water, along with fresh air, was the orthodox medical science of ancient Greece, Rome and Egypt.

2. In all ancient religions pure water was used for the purification of the body, and was referred to as "holy" because it did heal the body.

3. The Greeks reached a standard of clear thinking and physical perfection that has never been surpassed. The quality of their drinking water was the most important factor in the Greek way of life.

4. The absorption and release of carbon dioxide by the world's waters is used by Mother Nature to control the balance of gasses in our atmosphere.

5. Plants live on the food they make themselves from water, sunlight, carbon dioxide, and inorganic minerals. Animals and man are subject to the organic laws of nature.

6. Almost every early civilization was born and cradled on the banks of one of the Earth's great rivers.

7. The body's temperature is controlled through water.

8. The body could survive no more than three days without water.

9. Your brain is composed of approximately 15,000,000,000 powerful brain cells that are at least 70'% water.

10. Approximately 92% of the blood is composed of water.

11. The body is able to create a portion of its own distilled water when it oxidizes sugars, fats and proteins.

12. Next to oxygen water is the substance we need the most and suspect the least.

13. There are several different types of water: rainwater, snow water, rainwater, boiled water, hard water, soft water, tap water, deionized water, filtered

water, heavy water, glacier water and distilled water.

14. Approximately 15 - 17% of the total water in the body is stored in the muscles, another 10 - 15"% in the skin.

15. The average adult body contains approximately 45 quarts of water.

16. In a lifetime the average person consumes enough inorganic minerals to form a full sized stone statue of himself.

17. An extremely important function of water is flushing out toxins and excess salt from the body.

18. The body stores the chemicals in tap water in the arteries, veins, joints and vital organs.

19. Only pure water in conjunction with high zeta potential colloids helps to restore the functional integrity of the body.

20. Water softeners remove some of the hard minerals from water but add salt in their place.

21. Water has the capability of penetrating through a membrane into water of a denser quality. This is known as the law of osmosis.

22. The previous best way of completely cleansing the human body and nourishing the cells was by the internal use of the purest water available. We now know that the best way to cleanse the body is through the use of pure water to which high zeta potential colloids have been added.

This is the story of scientific intrigue. Nearly a century ago, the Father of Fluid Dynamics, Dr. Henri Coanda, began a search for the secret of living water—the legendary Fountain of Youth. This quest took Dr. Coanda all over the world. He traveled to remote mountain valleys where people live to be over 100 years old and yet remain in vibrant youthful health. A few of these places include Hunzaland in the Karakorum Mountains of Tibet, the Vilcabamba of Ecuador, and the country of Georgia in the Soviet Union. In all these places the centenarians attribute their good health to the special cloudy colloidal water they drink. When Dr. Coanda was 85 years old he passed the quest to 17 year-old Patrick Flanagan.

Thus began Dr. Flanagan's personal quest. After 14 years of research he had the answer. The key to long life was somehow contained in the structure of water.

In this book, Dr. Patrick Flanagan and his wife and co-researcher, Gael Crystal Flanagan reveal how they discovered the secret of Hunza water and thus fulfilled the quest.

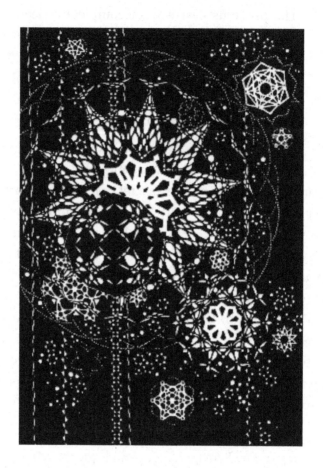

The illustration is a depiction of a crystal fountain. This design was made by Claude Bragdon, author, architect and mystic.

The design was originally published in the 1932 edition of Bragdon's book, The Frozen Fountain, published by Alfred A. Knopf.

Made in the USA
Middletown, DE
17 May 2021